BOOKS BY JOHN L. LOVE

Factuality

Mind Over Matter

Spiritually Connected

Surviving Our Lowest Point

For The Love Of Pets

From Legends To Legacy

Karma Sutra From A Master Seducer

Seven Times The Deadly Sinner

Business Is Business, No Skin Color Required

Guardian The Ghetto Hero

MIND
OVER
MATTER

By John L. Love

MIND OVER MATTER

MIND
OVER
MATTER

A Self-Help Guide Towards Unlocking The True Power Of
The Mind & Body

By John L. Love

POWER LEVEL LIMIT!

True Power is REAL!
Knowing how to unleash it is the hard part. In this book I teach you how to dig deep into your body as well as your mind to find it. Helping you unleash your hidden abilities as humans is simple if you just train the right parts of your body. I know this because I spent years training my body to overcome many different obstacles that most doctors said wasn't possible. I took the human body & made it do things that seemed impossible (By Eyesight) but not by (Physics). Throughout this book, you'll have the opportunity to train certain body parts in ways you never dreamed of, in addition to this; you'll be unleashing your ultimate human inner power.

John Lee Love
Minneapolis, Minnesota
June 2016

Index Glossary

WHAT IS POWER/
UNDERSTANDING
TRUE POWER

There are many definitions & ways of thinking about the term "POWER"

The first way people think of power has to do with "CONTROL", now this type of power has to do with controlling resources, influence, strength, political control, energy/ electricity ect. But in this book, I teach how to "Unleash" your TRUE POWER as a human being!!!

The power I teach has to do with, the ability to get your BODY to do things it would NOT normally do!

Today we go beyond that relatively vague & simple definition & look more closely at the FACTORS which make someone do something he or she would not normally do. As humans, we LIMIT ourselves to think that the human body cannot SURPASS its normal limits; which is not true at all, seeing that there are amazing body builders, & psychics walking the earth daily!!

That's just proof of how far our human minds, as well as bodies can go!

We as humans can exceed any limit the body will allow. Now im not saying we can shoot fire or breath souls, naw im personally saying there are substantial ways to push the body to run, jump, dodge, throw, withstand, dish-out different types of speeds as well as strength. But just like with anything else, I am here to teach you exactly how to build up this power, along with mastering its natural abilities. Throughout this book I will take you step-by-step towards surpassing your normal human abilities, & unleashing your true power!.

MASTERING
THE HUMAN
BRAIN

Now the first step to mastering the human body is simply the brain. The way we think, versus how we act all plays a significant part of our human brain!
 Knowing what to do, comes from understanding how to do it. In other words; we first need to understand, before we can do. Thus taking us back to the beginning of this, which is understanding the human brain.

Now to understand what the body is capable of doing, one must first understand what the brain will allow the body to do. When it comes to our brains, ill state ONLY FACTS!
These facts will allow you to master what your brain is capable of doing which will allow you to unleash your TRUE INNER POWER from within your BODY.
On this page as well as the following pages, ill state the facts.

No Pain:
There are no pain receptors in the brain, so the brain can feel NO PAIN.

Brain Growth:
Starting from the womb, "Fetal Brain" development begins to grow at birth which then continues to grow 18 more years!.

Cerebral Cortex:
The cerebral cortex grows "Thicker" as you learn to use it.

New Neurons:
Humans continue to make new neurons throughout life in response to mental activity.

Read Aloud:
Reading aloud & talking often to a young child promotes brain development.

Emotions:
The capacity for such emotions as joy, happiness, fear, & shyness are already developed at birth. The specific types of nurturing a child receive shapes how these emotions are developed.

First Sense:
The first sense to develop while in "Utero" is the sense of touch. The lips & cheeks can experience touch at about 8 weeks, & the rest of the body around 12 weeks.

Child Abuse:
Studies have shown that child abuse can inhibit development of the brain & can permanently affect brain development.

Oxygen:
Your brain uses 20% of the total oxygen in your body.

Blood:
As with oxygen, your brain uses 20% of the blood circulating in your body.

Unconsciousness:
If your brain loses blood for 8 to 10 seconds, you will lose consciousness.

Speed:
Information can be processed as slowly as (0.5 meters/sec) or as fast as (120 meters/sec) (about 268 miles/hr).

Wattage:
While awake, your brain generates between (10 & 23 watts) of power- or enough energy to power a light bulb.

Yawns:
It is thought that a yawn works to send more oxygen to the brain, therefore working to cool it down & wake it up.

Neocortex:
The Neocortex makes up about 76% of the human brain & is responsible for language & consciousness.

10%:
The "old saying" human's only use 10% of their brains is NOT TRUE. Every part of the brain has a known function.

Brain Death:
The brain can live for (4 to 6 minutes) without oxygen, & then begins to die. No oxygen for (5 to 10 minutes) will result in permanent brain damage.

Highest Temperature:
The next time you get a fever, keep in mind that the "Highest Temperature" ever recorded was (115.7) degrees- & the man survived.

Stress:
Excessive stress has shown to alter brain cells, brain structure & brain function.

Love Hormones & Autism:
Oxytocin, one of the hormones responsible for triggering feelings of love in the brain, has shown some benefits to helping control repetitive behaviors in those with autism.

Food & Intelligence:
A study of one million students in New York showed that students who ate lunches that did not include artificial flavors, preservatives, & dyes did 14% better on (I.Q) tests than students who ate lunches with these additives.

Seafood:
Eating seafood at least one time every week had a (30%) lower occurrence of dementia.

Tickles:
You can't tickle yourself because your brain distinguished between unexpected external touch & your own touch.

Reading Faces:
Without any words, you may be able to determine if someone is in a good mood, is feeling sad, or is angry just by reading the face. A small in the brain called the amygdale is responsible for your ability to read someone else's face for clues to how they are feeling.

Pain & Gender:
Scientists have discovered that men & women's brains react differently to pain, which explains why they may perceive or discuss pain differently.

Cold:
Some people are more sensitive to cold & actually feel more cold pain associated with cold, this is due to certain channels that send cold information to the brain.

Scent & Memory:
Memories triggered by scent have a stronger emotional connection; therefore appear more intense than other memory triggers.

Anomia:
Anomia is the technical word for tip-of-the-tongue syndrome when you can almost remember a word, but it just won't quite come to you.

Sleep:
While you sleep at night may be the best time for your brain to consolidate all your memories from the day.

No Sleep:
It goes to follow lack of sleep may actually hurt your ability to create new memories.

Brain Waves:
Brain waves are more active while dreaming than when you are awake.

Color Or Black & White:
Some people (about 12%) dream ONLY in black & white while others dream in color.

Virtually Paralyzed:
While you sleep, your body produces a hormone that may prevent you from acting out your dreams, leaving you virtually paralyzed.

Snoring:
If you are snoring, you are not dreaming.

Symbolism:
Dreams almost NEVER represent what they ACTUALLY are. The unconscious mind strives to make connections with concepts you will understand, so dreams are largely symbolic representations.

Blinking:
Each time we blink, our brain kicks in & keeps things illuminated so the whole world doesn't go dark each time we blink (about 20,000 times a day).

Laughing:
Laughing at a joke is no simple task as it requires activity in five different areas of the brain.

Thoughts:
The average number of thoughts that humans are believed to experience each day is 70,000.

Yawns Are Contagious:
Ever notice that you yawned after someone around you did? Scientists believe this may be a response to an ancient social behavior for communication that humans still have. The reason why we feel tired after the yawn is because cavemen, who probably spoke this language, always appeared to be in a "tired" state. They moved in a tiredly way; this is our bodies way to reenact how they were as well as yawning/ speaking (their language) the way they did.

Cannibalism:
Humans carry genes that help protect the brain from prion diseases, or diseases contracted through eating human flesh.

90% of the facts that I have listed on these past several pages, are all facts that'll help your brain unleash its full power.

MASTERING
THE HUMAN
BODY

Once you master the "human brain" thinking process, you can
then master how the human body is affected by the human
brain thinking effects!

In other words; YOUR action, will cause a REACTION,
which leads to a chain of effects!

In Martial Arts, we do NOT just punch & kick in ANY
direction. We are very precise when we attack. We calculate
EVERY POSSIBLE MOVE! From the way you breathe, on
down to the way you dress. Everything about YOU gets
calculated!

     & every calculation equals an EXECUTION! Nothing
is left to chance. In this section of the book, I'll teach you how
to master the human body, body parts. Knowing the body
parts will save you time as well as effort when in any fight.

The best fighters in the world studied the human body. They
never only learned how to throw a punch or a kick. Mastering
the human body was ALWAYS FIRST!

     This is the same concept i live by as well as teach daily.
On the next following pages, I'll explain how to "Pressure
Point"

Pressure points are a "Mastery" of art as well as skill. It takes
great "precision" as well as aim. If done correctly, it can be a
deadly finisher in any fight. But if done poorly, then it could
end up fatal....probably for you! Or it can leave your opponent
in a bad condition or worse. Remember if done correctly, it'll
leave your opponent paralyzed just the way you want them,
but first you have to master it.

Knowing where & when to strike the body is crucial. Mastery of this skill is keen to ending any fight in record time.
This diagram displays some common pressure points to try.

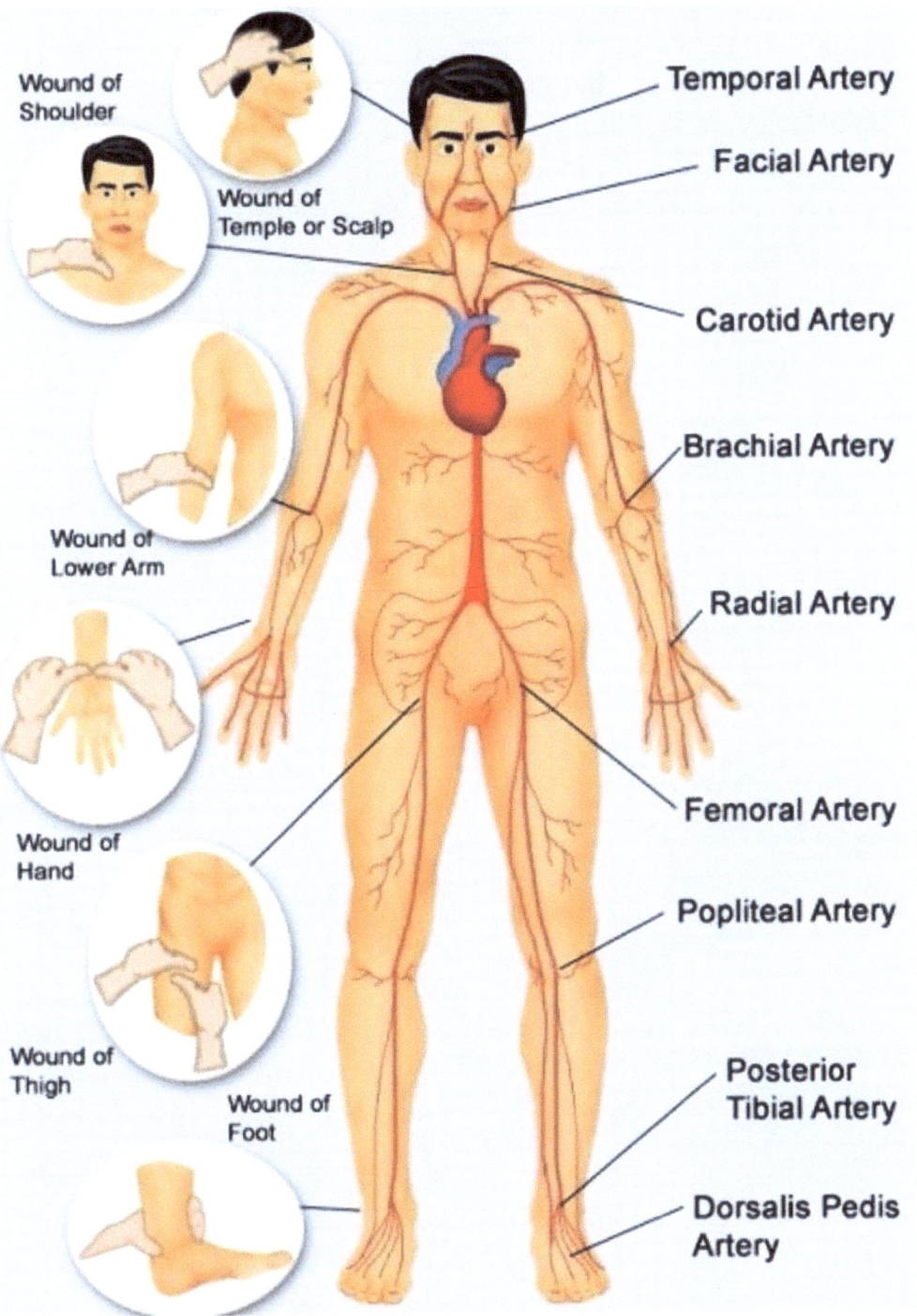

Wound of Shoulder

Wound of Temple or Scalp

Wound of Lower Arm

Wound of Hand

Wound of Thigh

Wound of Foot

Temporal Artery

Facial Artery

Carotid Artery

Brachial Artery

Radial Artery

Femoral Artery

Popliteal Artery

Posterior Tibial Artery

Dorsalis Pedis Artery

The pressure points (Name Labels) on this page are blurry but that's ok. You don't need to really know the name of the striking place; you only need to know if you really wanna know. But in this case you don't need to know. Knowing how the spot looks is all that matters.

Below in the diagram you'll notice the pressure points that affect you, is colored (bright-red) so you know the parts is being cut-off from blood circulation. Remember the more pressure you apply the more blood circulation you cut-off!

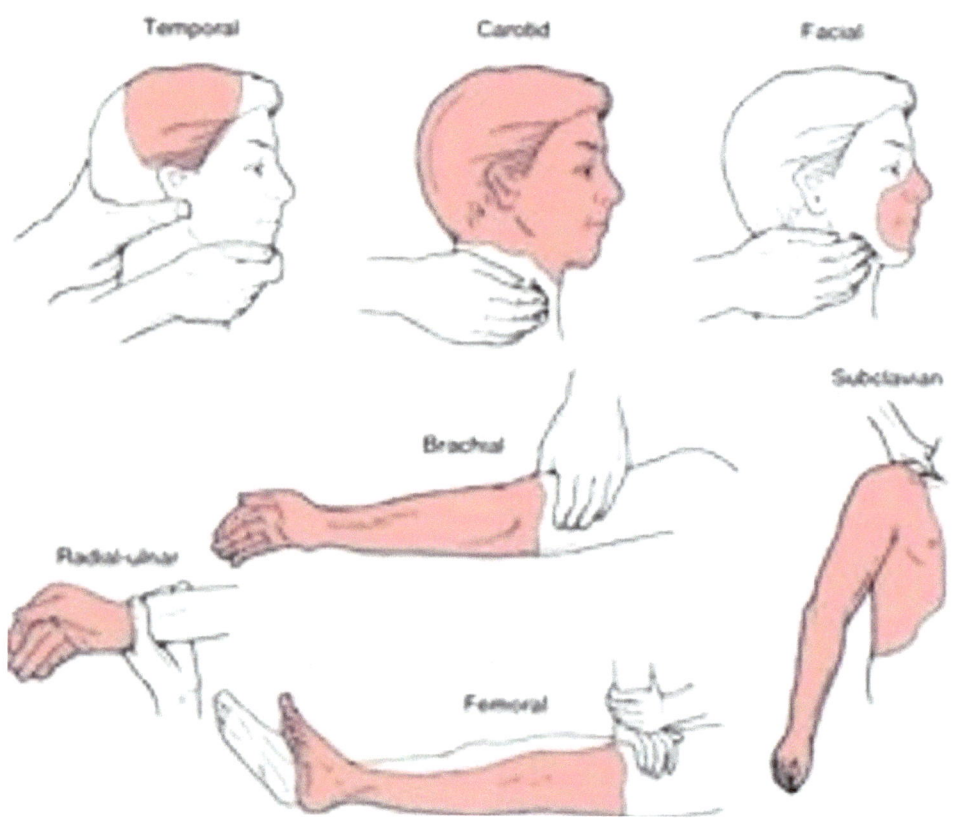

The best & easiest way to learn pressure points is to practice on yourself for nonstop learning. This way, you can feel the pressure & how much to apply to your opponent.

Always remember: Pressure points DON'T win FIGHTS! They only slow down or temporarily disable your opponent. You'll always need to add punches as well as kicks.

When it comes to mastering pressure points, speed is key to this technique. Without speed, you'll NEVER catch your opponent off guard!

As a matter of fact; later on in this book I'll teach you how to build up the speed as well as hand technique so you can execute every attack with keen precision!!

But for now, just keep in mind speed is always the way to go in any technique when it comes to fighting. Remember with pressure points, one needs to practice often to master it.

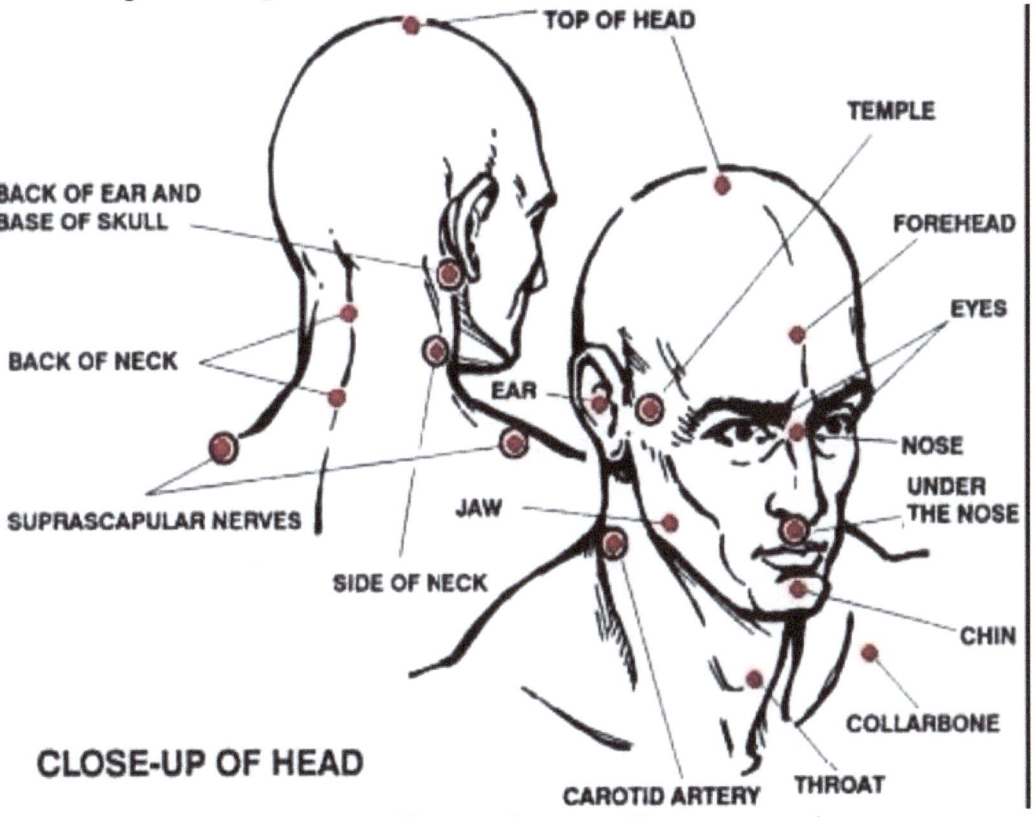

CLOSE-UP OF HEAD

Practice slowly as well as often until you get the pressure point placement down. Then use all the speed & intensity that you can. Keep noted: you fight how you practice!

If you practice slow & sloppy, that's how you'll fight & you probably won't last long. & if your focus is on speed, breathe normally (Bak Mei Kung Fu). Your arms can move faster than your lungs, while controlled breathing etc.

The traditional definition of a pressure point is a point that, when pressure is applied, produces crippling pain. This is learnt in a Chinese martial art called "Dim Mak" based on acupuncture pressure points, but this art is very restricted & needs understanding of Chinese acupuncture points. Because of this I can only provide information on fragile areas that we'll call "Vulnerable Points".

This is used to exploit a weakness or vulnerability in the human body to gain an advantage over an opponent. When using these pressure points one must be particularly careful as it is easy to kill someone accidentally, such as a friend or even an enemy. Below as well as the following pages I explain the different areas of pressure points as well as where to attack them.

Vulnerable Areas:

These are commonly known as pressure points. The points include the eyes, the groin, the shins, etc.

The Forehead:

Striking the "flat" of the forehead forces the head back with little resistance & will actually rock the brain within the skull, causing a concussion, or worse.

Temples:

The temples are the thinnest part of the cranium, so a good blow here (one-knuckle punch is ideal) can cause concussion, hemorrhaging, or even death. Do NOT strike a training partner with this move!.

Look For The Collar Bone:

Once located, jab your fingers behind bone & force to the ground (this needs to be performed within about ¼ second in an actual assault).

Neck/Sleeper:

This is another more obvious pressure point but is very complicated in application. Get behind your assailant & wrap one arm around his neck, using your "Radius" (Forearm Bone), apply pressure to the "External Carotid Artery" (just to the side of the throat where you feel your pulse beating), slowly lowering them to the ground as you do so. You can increase the pressure by pulling your arm toward you with the other arm, & breathing in as you do, puffing up your chest. You can also place the hand of the squeezing arm in the elbow of the other arm & push the head/neck forward with that other arm. If they show no signs of weakening a sharp blow to the back of the head will disorientate them giving you a chance to run.

The Throat:

The easiest way to strike is probably with a "Knife Hand" (Karate Chop) turned upside down. A fist will have trouble fitting between the jaw & collarbone. You can also grab & squeeze the throat, & even give it a good yank to dislocate it & make breathing impossible. That is, of course, quite lethal & should be used only as a last resort when there is no other alternative.

Jaw Zone:

Under the jaw; grab the neck on the front & reach under the jaw. Squeeze while pressing upward.

Support the head with one hand. With the other, follow the jaw line to the highest point, just under the ear, where it meets the bump in your skull. Apply pressure inward & upward towards your ear. This is painful & makes speaking very difficult. If possible, a person will try to move away from it, hence the supporting hand. A single-knuckle punch (the second middle finger knuckle) to this spot could dislocate the jaw.

Forearm/Crevice:

The crevice of your forearm is made entirely of muscles & tendons, so there's lots to work with. Grab the elbow with your thumb on top. Place your fingers on the back of the elbow for a good grip. Squeeze the tip of your thumb toward the tips of your index or middle finger. You have to reinforce the thumb with your fingers, or you'll lose leverage. Press the thumb into the middle of crevice, into either side of the crevice, or into the lump on the outer forearm formed when you make a fist (the brachioradialis). Experiment with this one. It can be rather tricky.

Back Of The Hand:

If you are grabbed, look directly at the hand of your assailant, & with either a regular or "Single-Knuckle" punch, strike the bones in the back of the hand. When practicing with a partner, give it one good shot, so you're not doing it all day. It only hurts for a minute.

Pinch The Fingers For A Simple Defense:

When punches are thrown, catch one in your armpit & lock down tight. Grab the upper inner part of the elbow joint- this needs to be done fast. Pinch down hard one finger on each side. This causes excruciating pain & will make your opponent's arm feel like it's breaking.

Torso Region:

"Sternum" strike with a single-knuckle to the bone in the middle of the chest. It has no muscle & never much fat, so it is very vulnerable, & if struck properly can break in two down the middle. You can also strike the pectorals like this. Edit; breaking the sternum can cause a punctured lung or worse. Be very careful with this & do not practice on friends.

Solar Plexus:

This is a bundle of nerves deep within the center of the "Abdomen", though to be responsible for the physical feelings of deep emotions. By striking the area just below the sternum, where the ribs join on the front of the abdomen, you affect this bundle of nerves & cause the "Diaphragm" (breathing muscle) to contract violently. This is "Knocking the wind out" of someone. It's a very easy target. This can be countered by flexing the abs quickly at the time of impact, which is accomplished by breathing out or yelling (Kiai).

Love Handles:

Place your hand flat on the side of the abdomen, between the ribs & hips. Roll your fingers in toward your palms. Do not pinch. Pinching does next to nothing. This will on any body type.

Ribs:

The ribs have very little covering, regardless of the body type, & only thin muscle between them. To break them, raise the arm to extend them, reducing their ability to reinforce each other, & step towards them when you strike. A palm-down knife hand works very well for this. Uppercuts also work for this as they seem to be designed to get right up under the arm, which is what you're aiming for. The rib areas protected by the muscles of the chest or back will not be easily broken, if at all. The lowest ribs connect only to the spine & so are especially vulnerable to breaking.

Feet:

Look down at the foot, & using your heel, raise your knee as high as you can, & stomp on the (arch of the foot) as hard as you can. Because of its structure, it can easily be broken. Do not strike the toes. It will hurt, but you certainly won't break anything.

Possible Therapeutic Uses:
If feeling drowsy or can't concentrate using both pointer fingers, apply pressure. Apply this pressure to temples, the flanks of the bridge of your nose &the corners of your eyes about (5mm) from the bridge of your nose.

Headaches Are A Pain:
Temporary relief or dulling of pain can be achieved by using the appropriate pressure point.
Front of head: massage both temples.
Middle/top of head: apply pressure to point just above ears.
Back of head: place both thumbs just behind ears & trace backwards until you find the point where your skull ends. Move another mm inwards & apply pressure.

Practice On Yourself & With A Friend:
Everybody is different & has different levels of pain tolerance. Where one point may be on you could be an inch to the left on someone else. Some don't feel at all. the more people you can practice with, the better you can be at approximating where a point should be & finding it when it's not there.

Practice Your Focus:
Always look directly at your target. If your eyes aren't there, your focus isn't.

Hone Your Techniques:
Key things to bear in mind when practicing include:
Use the tips of your fingers & thumbs for techniques using either. This works like a needle, focusing all the force into the very tip of your finger/thumb, multiplying the pressure per square inch (PSI). Keep your knees bent, at least a little, at all times. More-so when doing techniques. This gives you stability & power. If you're standing straight up, you're like an upright piece of wood, ready to be pushed right over.

FOODS
FOR
POWER

If you're looking for the "Fountain of youth", stop looking in your medicine cabinet & take a closer look into your pantry. What we put in our bodies affects everything from the size of our waistlines, the condition of our hearts, & yes-even how long we live.

In (Okinawa), Japan who are known to age more healthily & tend to live longer than most places in the world. Or the residents of the (San Blas Islands) who have incredibly low rates of heart disease. Or (Seventh Day Adventists) who live up to seven years longer than their neighbors, on average. What's food got to do with it? Well a lot.

So, to help you celebrate more birthdays, I rounded up some (Research-Backed) foods to add to your diet.
Below on this page as well as the following page, I listed a short list of foods to add to your diet.

Cranberries:
Love'em hate'em, these tart & somewhat bitter berries are good for you. Researchers found young fruit flies given cranberry extract lived 25 percent longer than those that weren't. & in even better news, middle age-aged & older fruit flies lived 30 percent longer!

Green Tea:

Besides boasting benefits like reduced risk of cancer & heart disease, the world's second most popular beverage was shown to reduce risk of death by up to 26 percent for those who consumed several cups a day.

Nuts:

People who snacked on a handful of nuts everyday were found to live longer than those who didn't, they also lived healthier lives with a lower chance of developing cancer, heart disease, & respiratory disease.

Salmon:

Smoked, baked, on a bagel, or in your sushi, you'll want to load up on the omega-3 rich fish. A diet rich in omega-3's could help preserve your telomeres, & slow down the aging process. Telomeres are the ends of your chromosomes that shrink with age.

Blueberries:

Often dubbed a "Super food" because of their high (Antioxidant) levels, blueberries & other foods rich in polyphenols can extend your life. Polyphenols can reduce your risk of death by 30 percent, the antioxidant has been shown to cut the risk of cancer & diabetes.

Whole Grains & Olive Oil:

Whole grains as well as olive oil increases lifespan by about 20 percent.

Wine:

Just half a glass of wine a day can help men live longer, light wine drinkers lives up to five years longer than those who did not drink at all. Red wine in particular is rich in antioxidants that help protect against heart disease.

TRAINING
WITH BODY
WEIGHTS

When it comes to weights & fighting, many people feel they have to only lift actual weights. Now this isn't as true as it may sound. Fighters…of many different sorts don't really lift weights. As a matter of fact; 99% of fighters don't lift weights. I only say this because lifting weights only makes the body "bulky" which in return slows down the fighters' movements the only type of weights fighters associate with is "body weights" as seen in the picture below, this is one type of punching weights that different cultures use for speed.

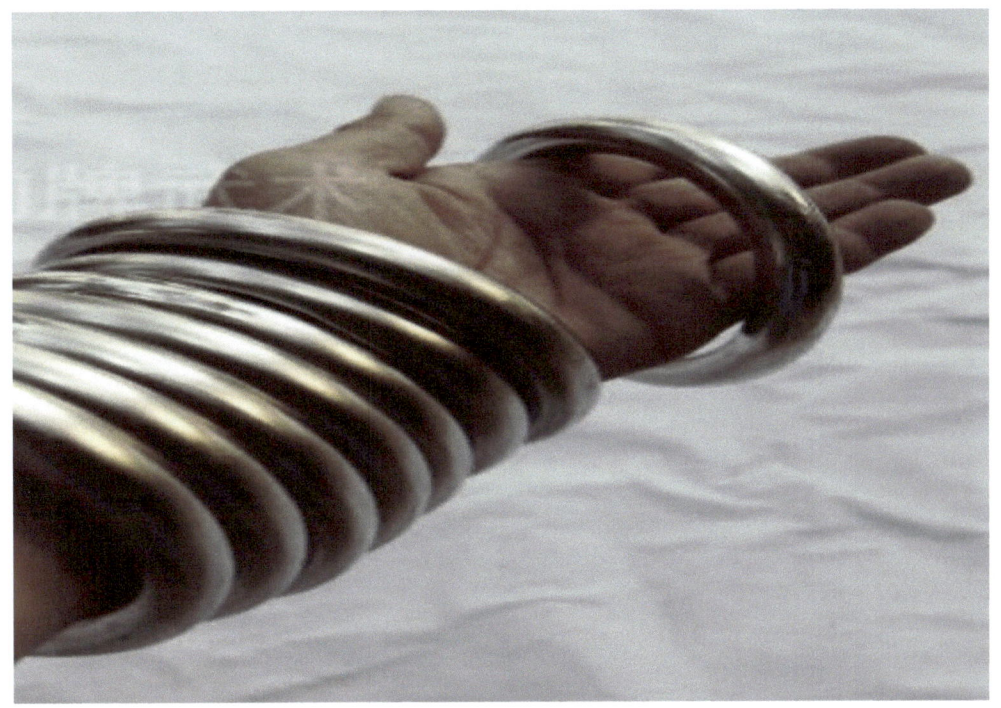

but if you are looking for a more "Traditional" style then these (Weighted) vest are some of the best choices.

In addition to these "vests" there is other weighted clothing that can be added to your training.

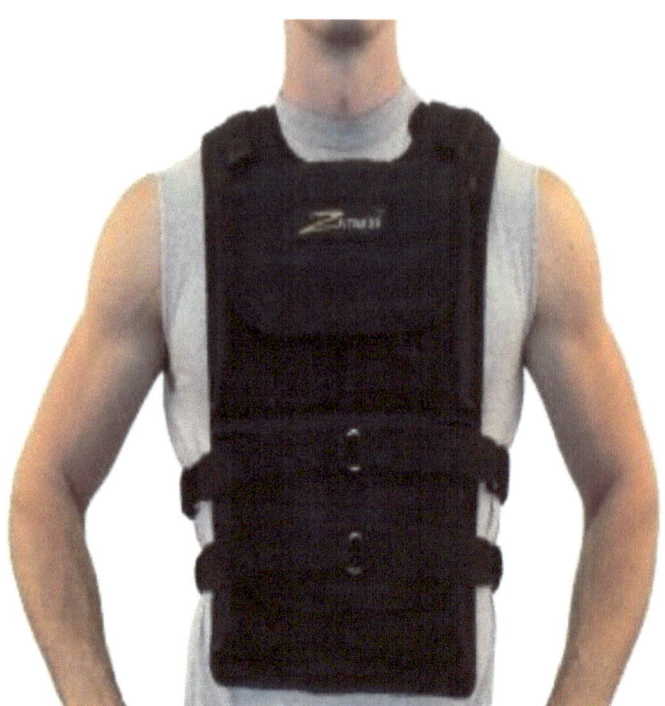

In this picture (Below) shows a weighted vest for women, there are other weighted clothing for children as well. When it comes to training, there is always something for everyone.

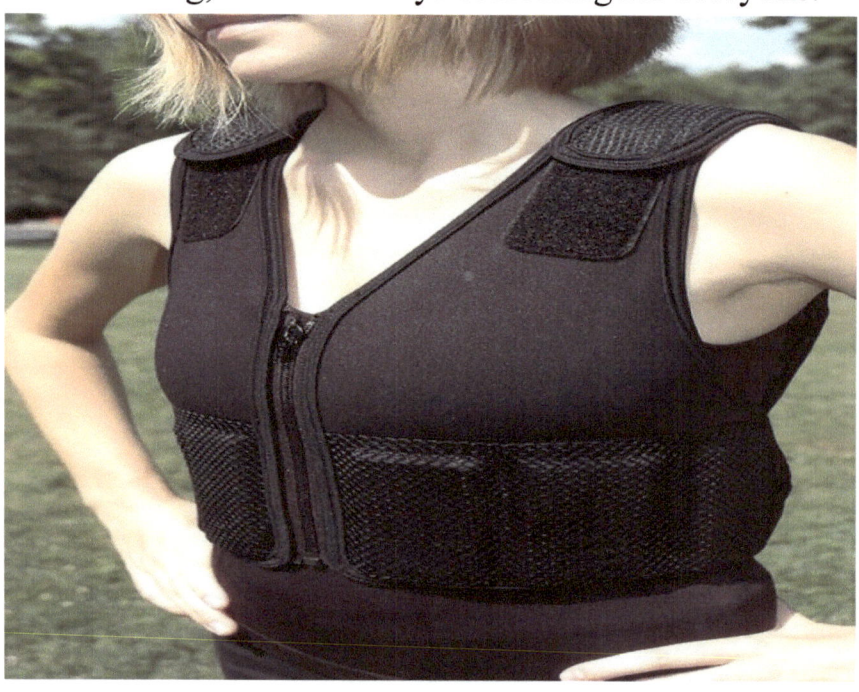

The best part about weighted gear that I personally love is that they come in different sizes to support your different body needs, as well as (Adjustable) weight pieces to help gradually build you up! Like in this image (Below) this weighted vest supports upper body, as well as (Sit-ups).

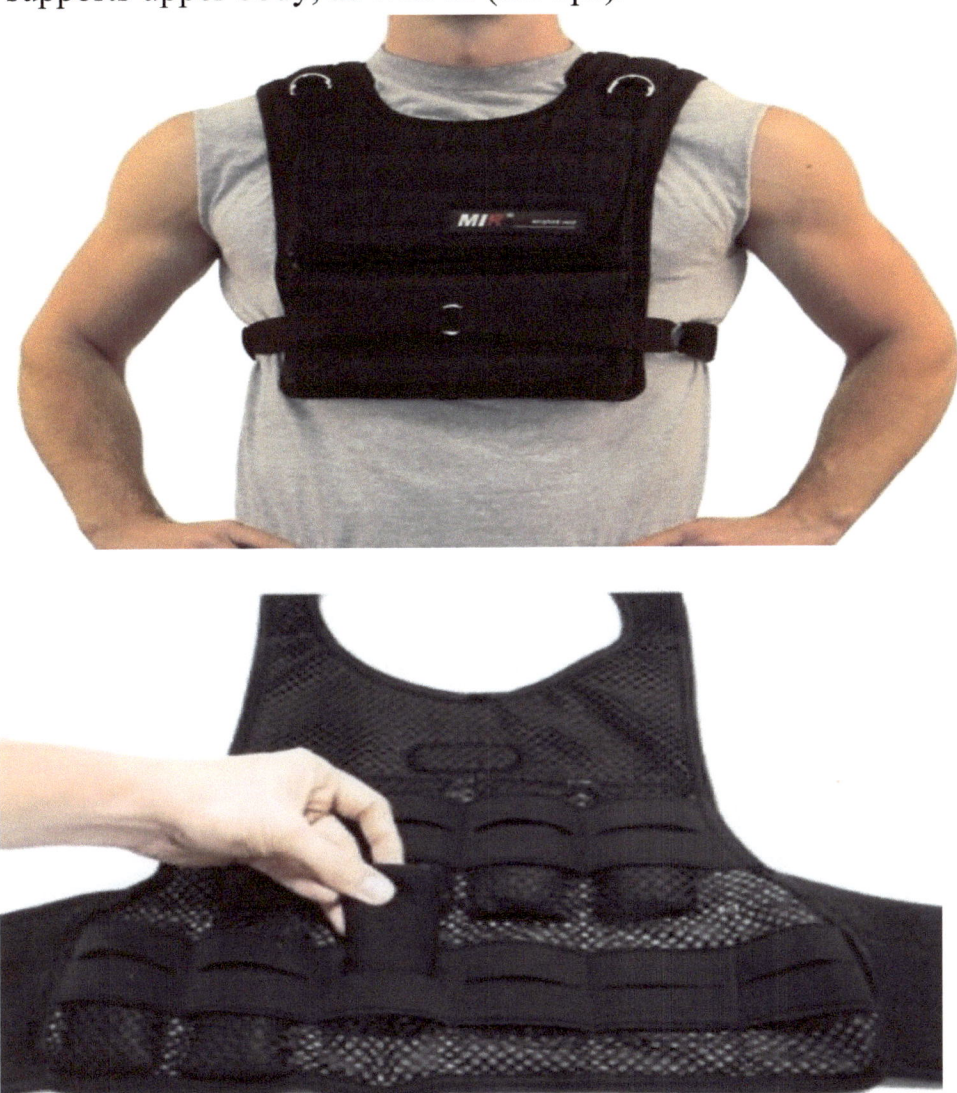

The (Vest) in this image shows how the weights can be adjusted to fit your body needs.

When it comes to weighted (Shorts) or pants; if you can find them. The (weights) are located in the "Bottom" section usually "above" the knee area. The only down-fall to this is the amount of weights they can carry.

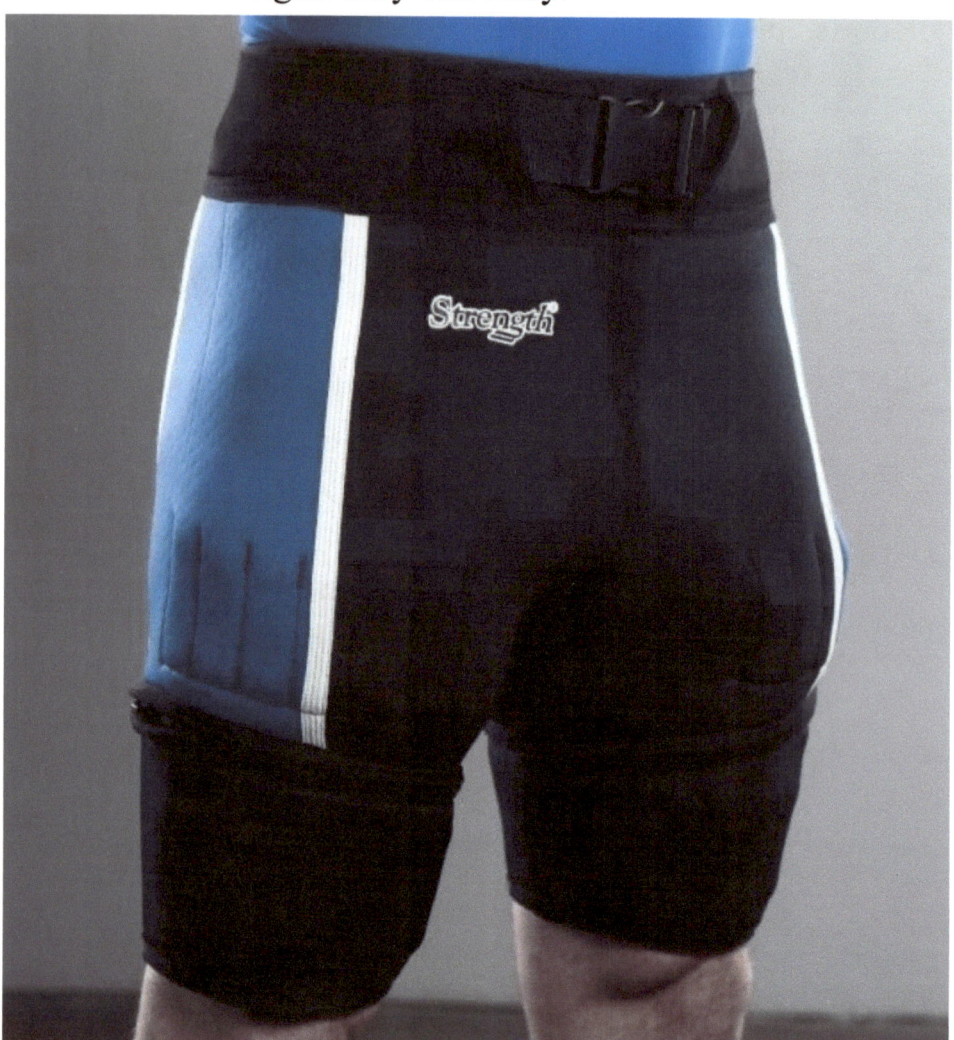

Like in the image (above) you can see the "zippers" on both legs. Those aren't pockets; those are where you would adjust your weights that are removable. The "lines" on the leg areas are different sections of weights; this shows the (Spacing) between the weights; as well as how many weights the shorts can carry at once. But there are other advanced weighted shorts that allows (more) weight carrying.

For instance, this particular pair of weighted shorts can hold twice as many weights as the previous pair, as well as provide extra movement performance!

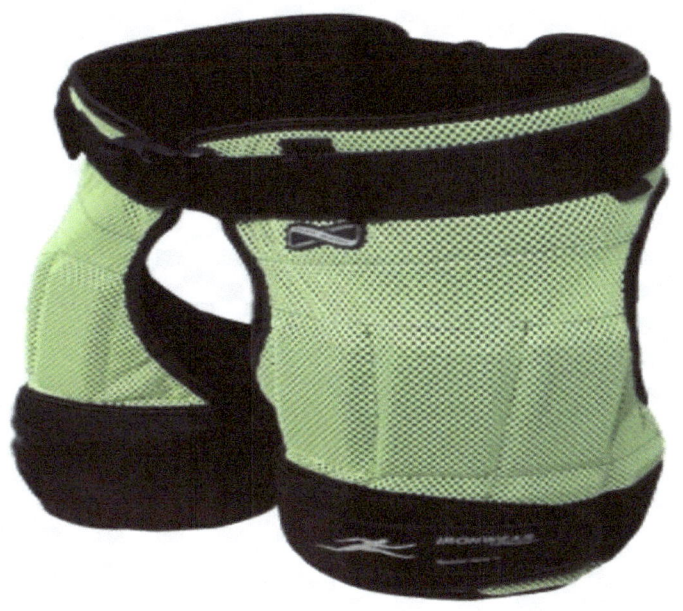

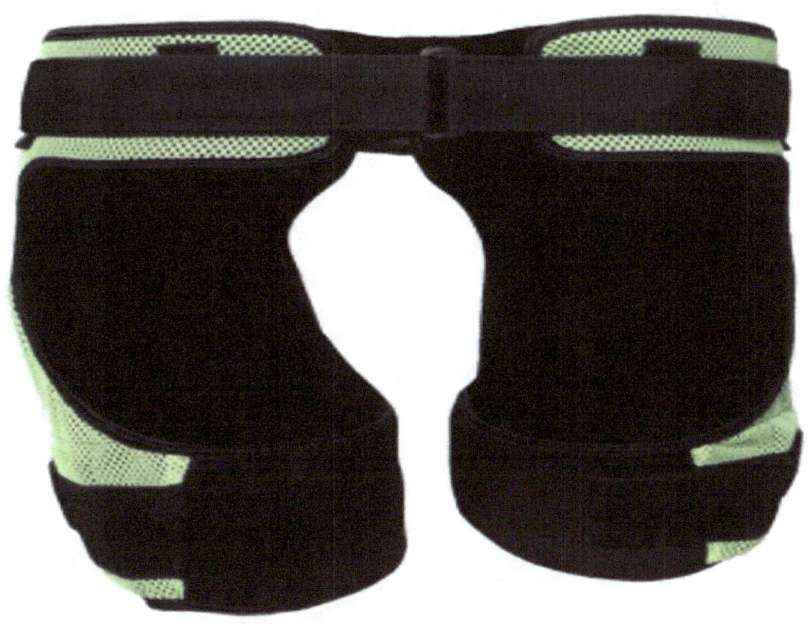

Next on the weighted gear list is the (feet) area of the body, yes the shoes. You can't fully train the body unless the whole body is getting the training. That's the only way one can unlock their full body power potential!

In the pictures (Below) are "slip-on" weights for your shoes.

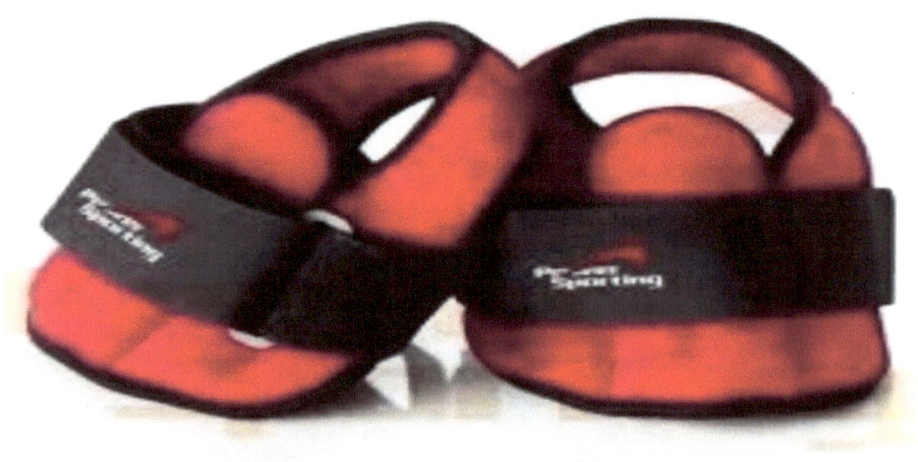

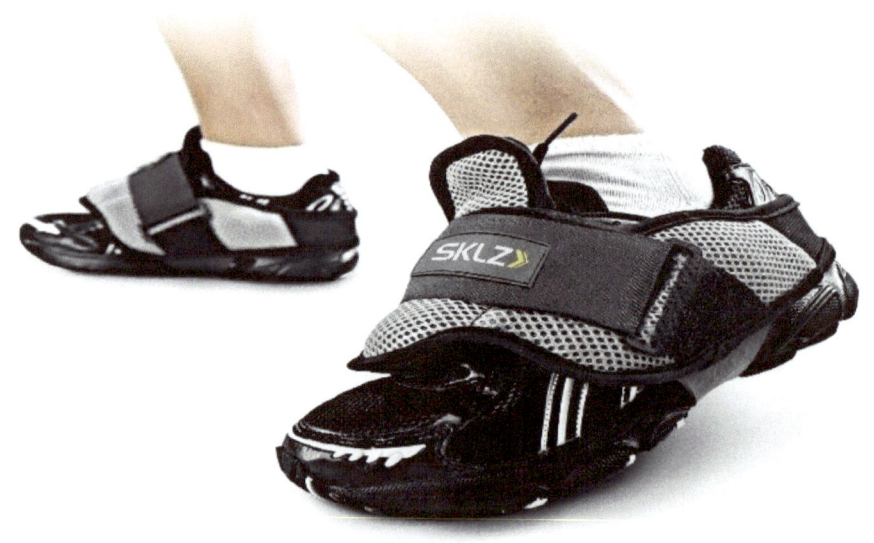

When it comes to (feet) weights, one can never go wrong. Feet weights provide that extra foot power one needs to execute deadly kicks; or if you are simply looking for increasing your speed. Weighted feet gear will provide all of that, giving you the advantage over any other opponent who never wore them.

But if you are like me, & you are looking for that ultimate (kick-ass) performance in training as a fighter, than you'll need a pair of these (Foot) shoes!

These are very pricey but worth every penny!!! These give you SUPERB leverage over ANY type of ground pavement...in addition to this; you can also wear the foot weights over these!

These are superb if you are a (Free-Runner) or a (Parkour) runner. These are also ideal for wall climbing, as well as rock climbing!

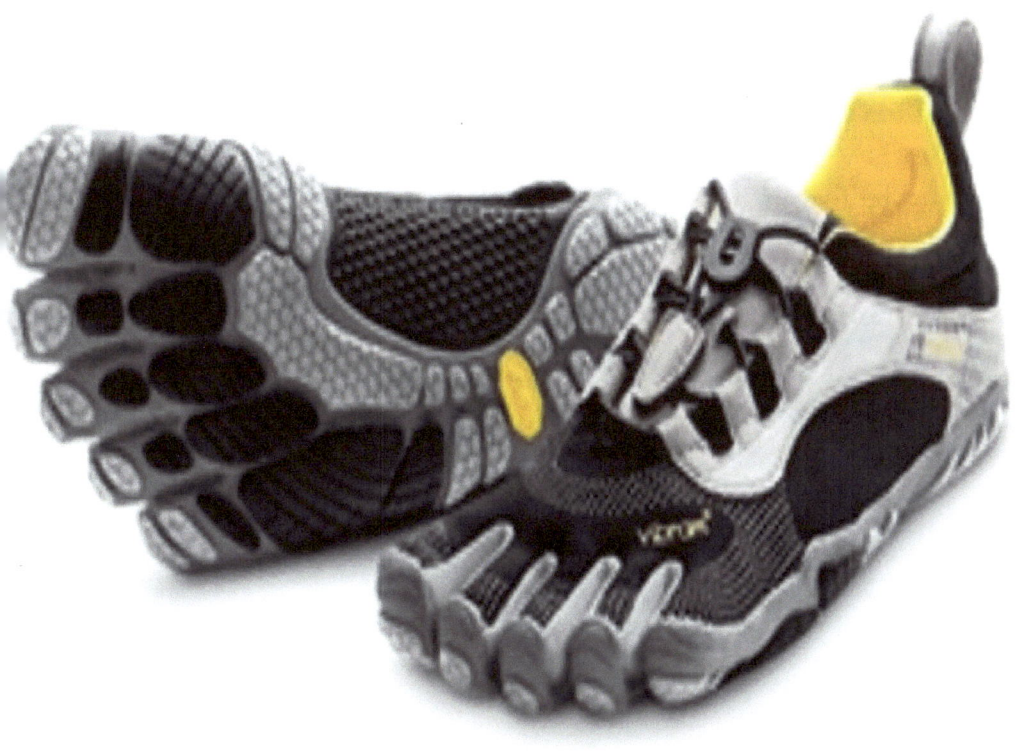

Despite all the weighted gear out there, I personally "pushed" my body beyond its normal limits!

I took weighted gear to another level & added it to my sleeping arrangements. I felt "why should I only wear weights?"

Better yet, "why can't I sleep in weights?"

Now you're probably thinking, why in the hell would someone want to sleep in body weights? Well to answer that question is simply because of my (insomnia) now how I deal with that is, I went out searching for ALL TYPES of weighted products, & I found a weighted blanket!!!

The weighted blanket keeps the body in a (Snug-Tight) position making one feel a safe-comfort feeling. Now this may sound weird to you, but try sleeping with a weighted blanket…you'll see the warmth comfort it brings as well as training the body at the same time!

The heavy weights it's made with, gives the body durability as well as speed. I swear after sleeping with this blanket, my speed increased by over 40%

& that's without wearing all the other body weights!!

Below is an image of what weighted blankets look like in case you or someone you know wants to buy one. They usually sell in online stores. So good-luck trying to find one in a regular store.

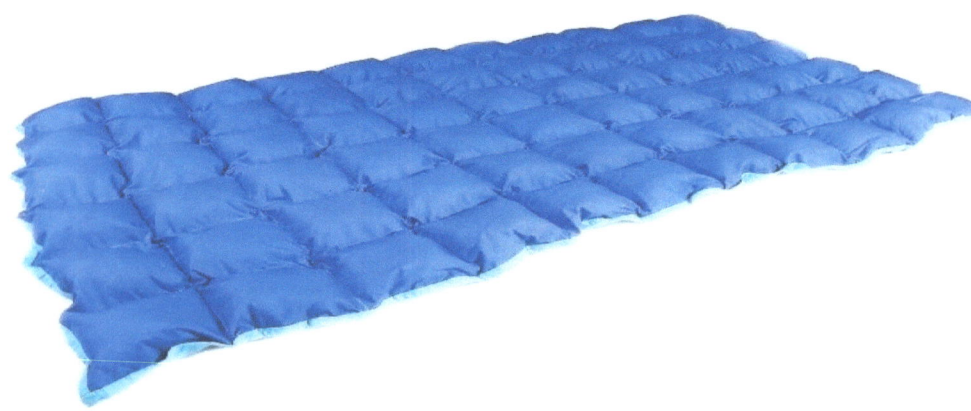

Just like with all the other weighted gear. Weighted blankets & any other weighted merchandise comes in both types of (sex) genders.

Another great thing about weighted gear is that you can personally add or create your own weights to add to them, just in case they are not heavy enough.

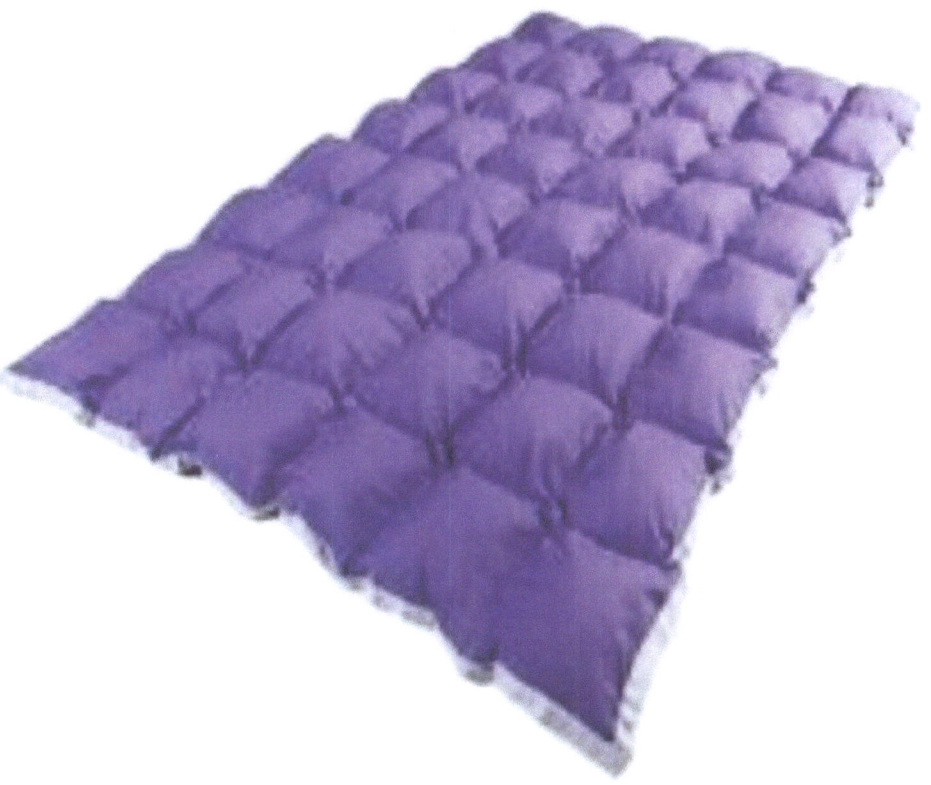

I personally added extra weights to all of my weighted gear. This gives me a substantial advantage in combat!

It also reshapes my body in a way that makes me extra durable to many attacks that my normal body could never endure. In addition to increasing my speed, my jumps, climbing, dodging, & counter attacking! All at once. & did I mention my strength? Wearing weights increases your lifting abilities as well; even my weighted blanket does this.

TRAINING
UNDER
WATER

When it comes to (weight training) under water plays a major part in this. This is simply because "water" well being under water, covers your whole body with weight. While regular weights can only cover certain parts of your body, which doesn't give you the maximum endurance. Water weight training also gives you (Hydration) something regular weights can't give you. Think about it. You're under water the whole time you are training, so there wouldn't be any need for you to break any sweat. Also, under water weight training also increases your ability to breath under water. This technique comes in handy in all situations; including breathing problems. It also allows you to learn to (calm) your heart pulse rate so you can focus more, this is what I like to call "deep water meditation" this is more of a (Ninja) technique which I personally mastered. This technique requires a lot of focus as well as overcoming "fear phobias" In addition to under water training, you'll be able to increase your speed, jump higher, run faster, maneuver quicker, along with hydrating your body & losing weight! As a simple warning: I advise you to start off slow... get the feel of the water...wherever you are. For me, I used a simple "indoor pool" Indoor pools work the best; just make sure it is empty of other people so you can train in peace. Also bring a water proof (stop-watch) to clock how long you can breathe under water. This is the only way to know if you are making breathing progress.

When it comes to under water training, any & every fighter who wanted to condition their bodies in the best way used this method; including the great champion (Muhammad Ali).
This method was introduced to me by the great Ali himself. Growing up I applied this method to (Kung Fu) & mastered the ways of the water. (Below) is a picture of Mr.Ali "water boxing"
This was one of his main ways of building his amazing endurance.

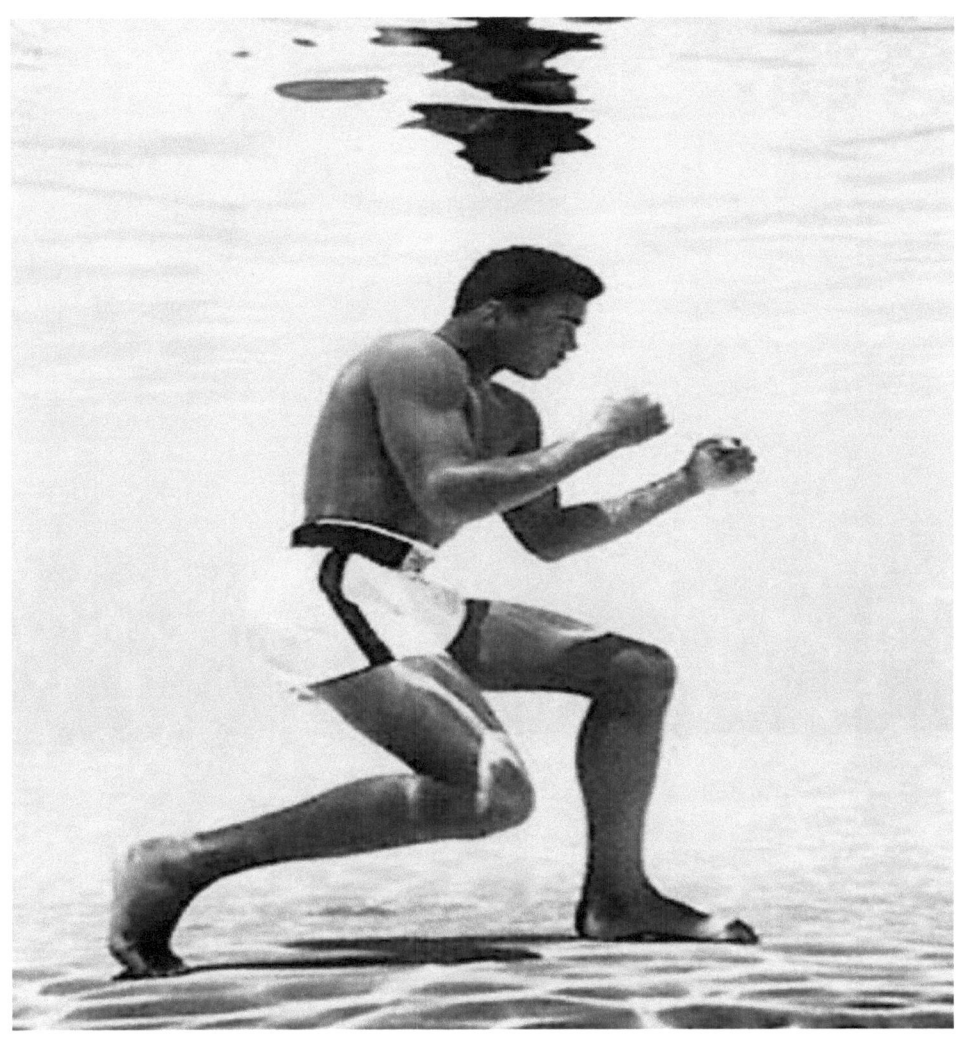

When training under water, you tend to put your (Mind over Matter) which means to focus your mind, over the extreme matters at hand. In this case, the water.

I say this because many people tend to go under water & instantly began to go into (panic) mode. They do this by thinking about how long they can breathe under water without drowning. In the image (Below) as you can see, the man in the image has weighted water shoes on, while he's holding his breath. This is what (Mind over Matter) is. It is simply defying one situation to overcome another. This is something you'll have to endure in order to unlock your true inner power to surpass your original human abilities.

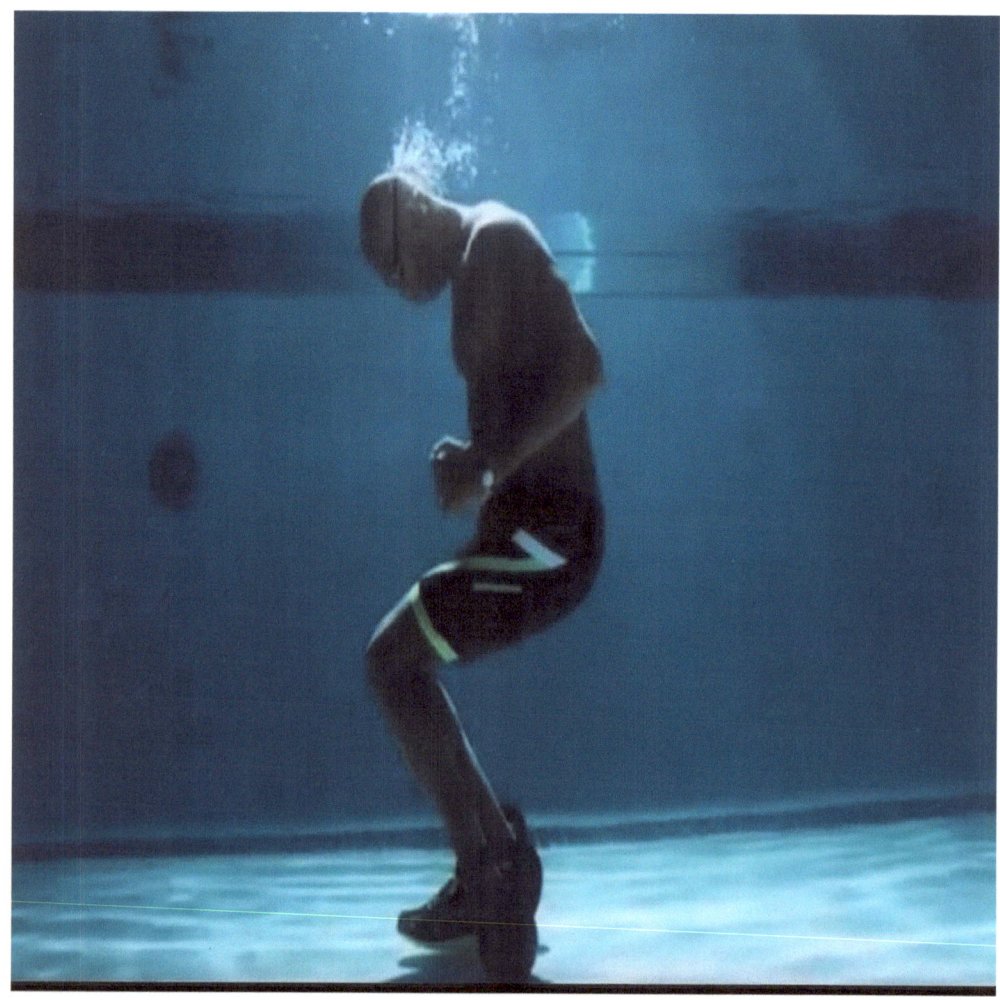

UNLOCKING
TRUE PUNCH
POWER

When it comes to the human body & unleashing its true power many fighters have the secret….but only one main fighter had surpassed that secret..& his name was (Bruce Lee) Master (Bruce Lee) to be exact. Bruce Lee was one of the first Martial Artist to push power passed its normal limits. In the (picture) below shows Master Bruce Lee showing that power through his (One-Arm two-Finger) push-ups! To perform this, one must first understand, as well as master (Mind over Matter) Besides Master Bruce Lee, I have also mastered this technique; Which in return allowed me to perform these push-ups.

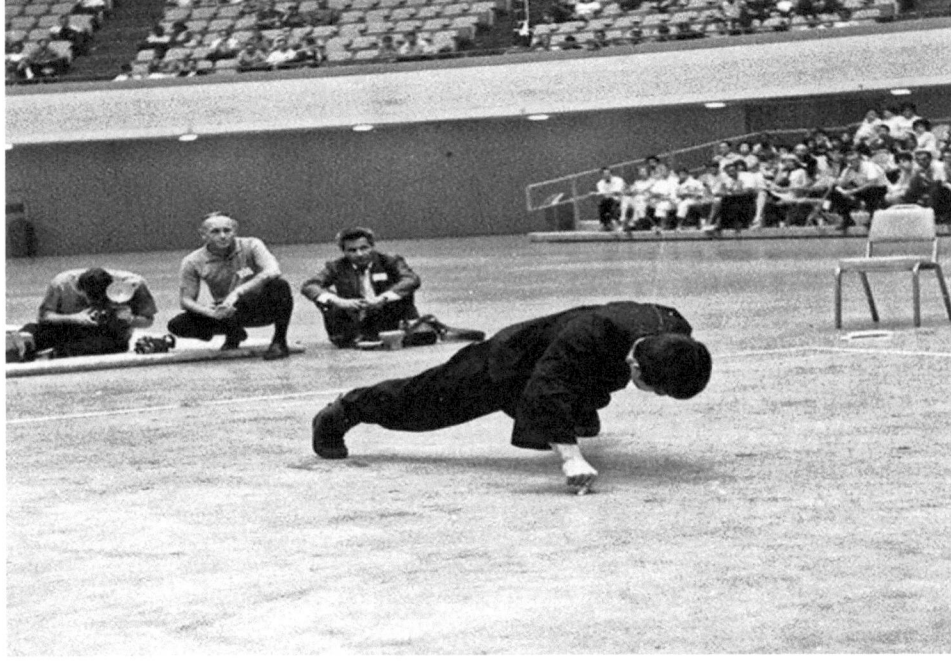

Because of this technique, I was unable to unlock the true power in myself to unleash powerful punches!!

Now the average human can punch basic objects & hurt themselves.

I learned to build up massive hand strength against painful objects 'to increase my fist strength. To do this I had to punch "steel" repeatedly, just simple small punching taps everyday to (Tenderize) my fist. Doing this gave my fists the advantage to hitting objects that are way harder than the human body. Just like in the picture (Below) I had to take a (cinderblock) like the one in the picture & punch it every day to build muscle strength.

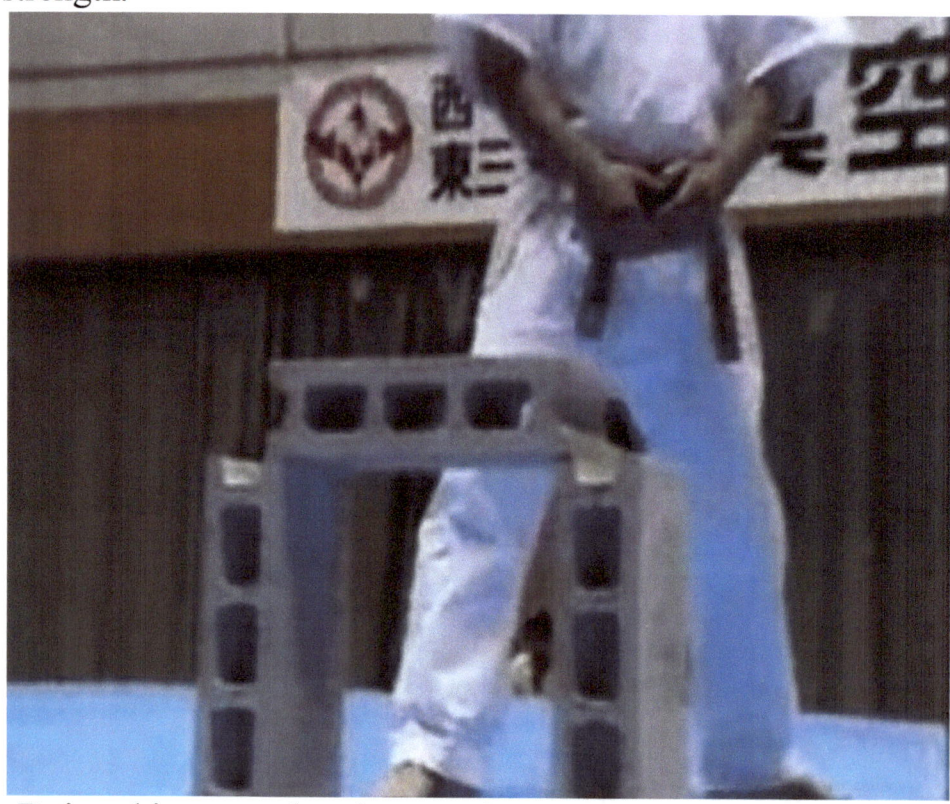

Doing this every day for months was enough to give me the ability to perform (One-Hitter-Quitters) also known as a (Knock-Out) punch! On the following pages I'll show you what true punch power looks like as well as what it takes to really push out that deadly "punch power".

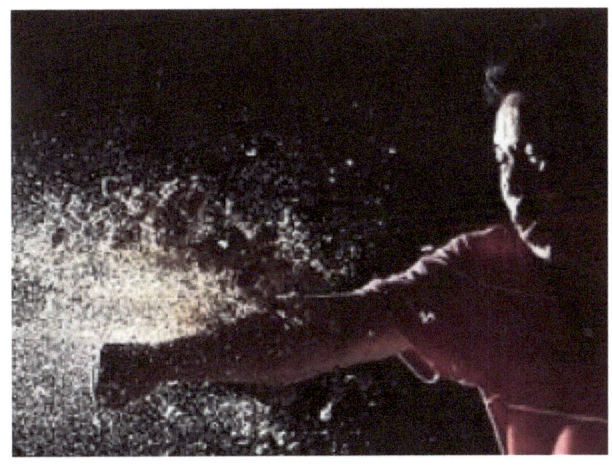

its punches like these that makes power more of a reality then "make-belief" I say this because the average human doesn't think he or she can perform such a punch. But as humans we are all capable of performing these types of punches, we just need practice on developing our fist enough to perform them.

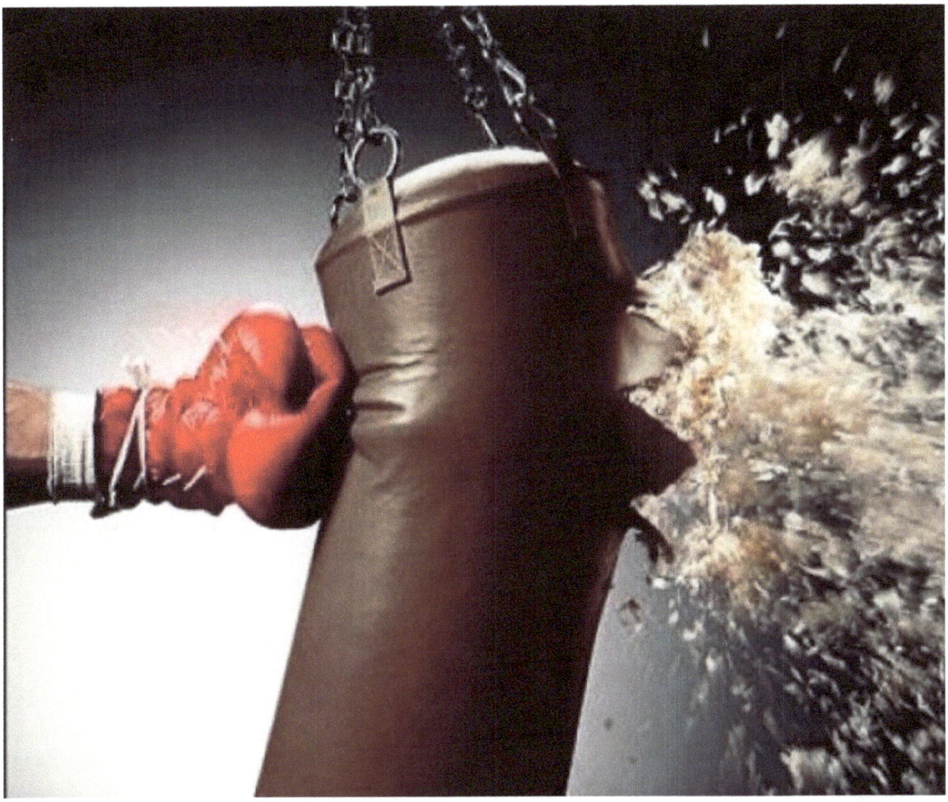

All these different types of power punches can be performed by certain ways of standing as well as positioning your body. On the following pages, I'll show & explain different types.

The first step in knowing how to punch in a (Powerful) explosive way, first one needs to learn how to make a fist the proper way. The way you position your fists, is the way your punch will be executed.

Good
Bad
Bad

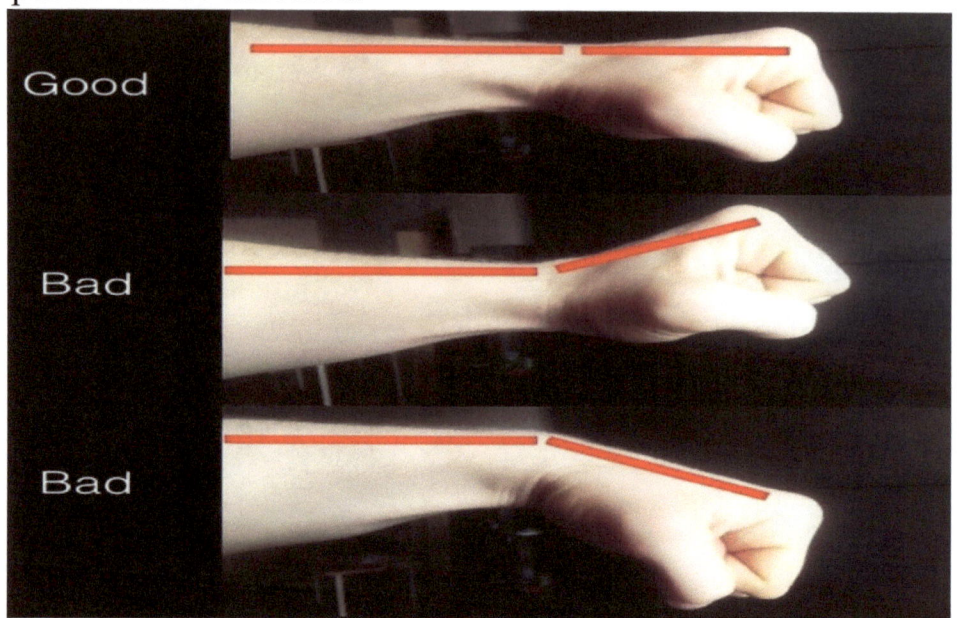

The (Bottom) image shows a basic punching stance

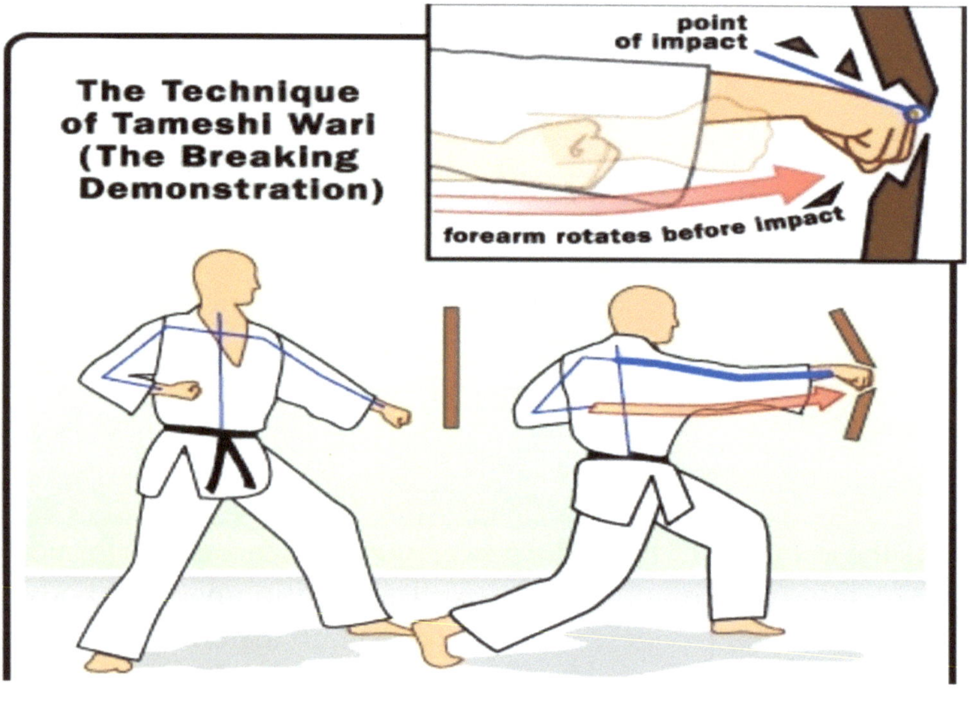

The Technique of Tameshi Wari (The Breaking Demonstration)
point of impact
forearm rotates before impact

Knowing how to position your fists isn't enough. To unleash your ultimate power, one has to master how to "Cuff" their thumb over their (First two) fingers. While straightening their wrist. If your "wrist" isn't straight, then you'll break your fist!

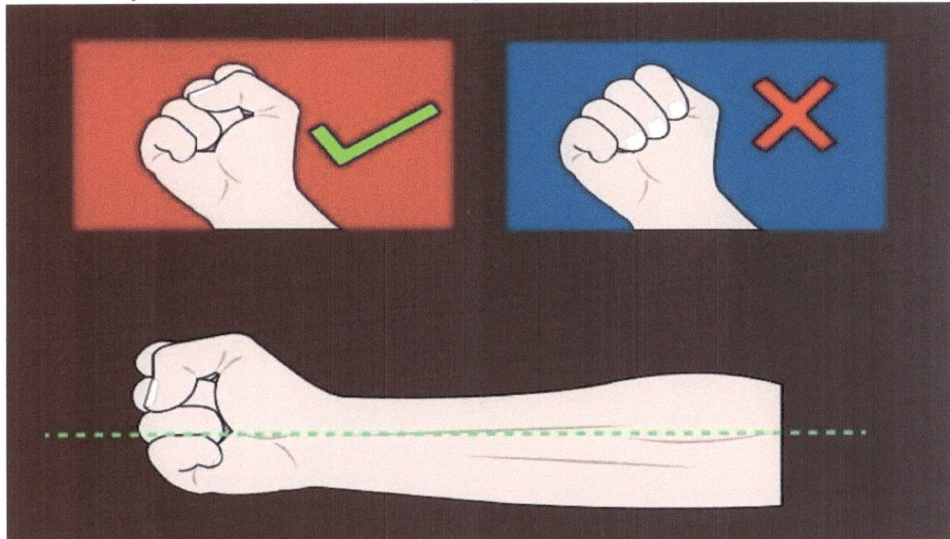

in addition to this, one must have confidents in the mastery of their punch, believing in your attacks is one way to help execute them properly; like in the image (Below) that is a basic example of what our fists can do with the power we have.

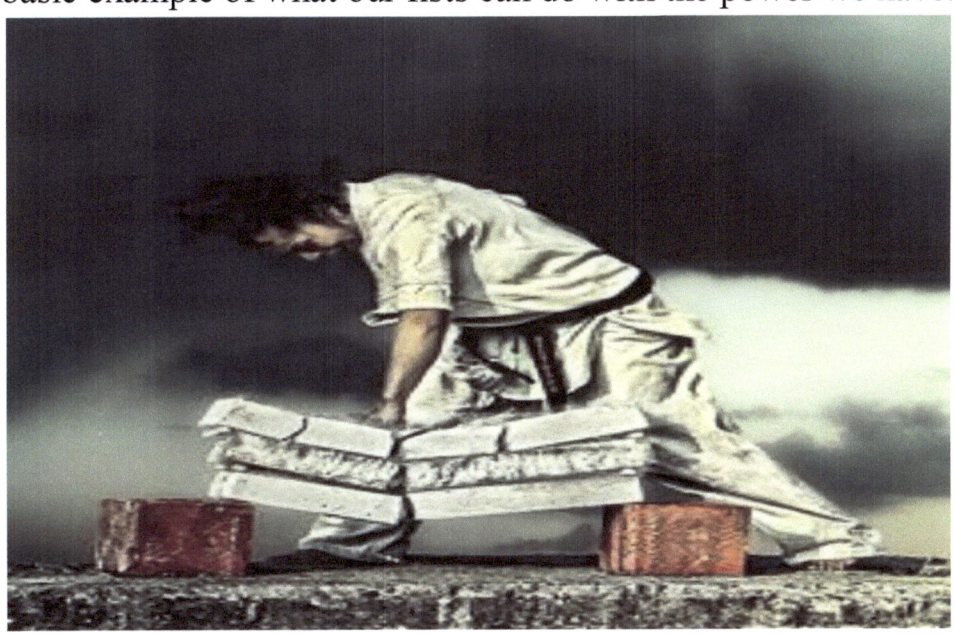

Our basic power comes from our stance, the stance you choose determines the amount of power you "dish" out. Using (Gravity) to unleash power is another key to letting your true power flow.

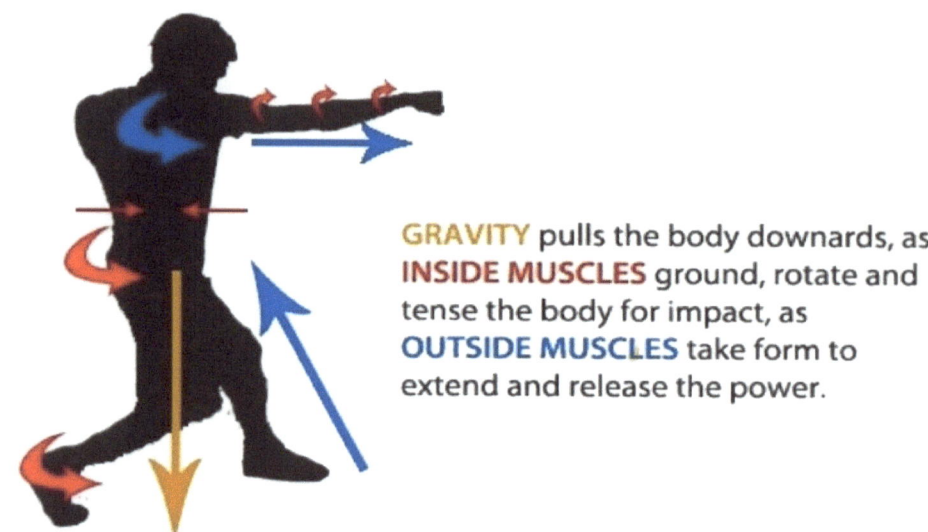

GRAVITY pulls the body downwards, as INSIDE MUSCLES ground, rotate and tense the body for impact, as OUTSIDE MUSCLES take form to extend and release the power.

Just like in the image (Below) using gravity can help in maneuvering ones power in many different ways.

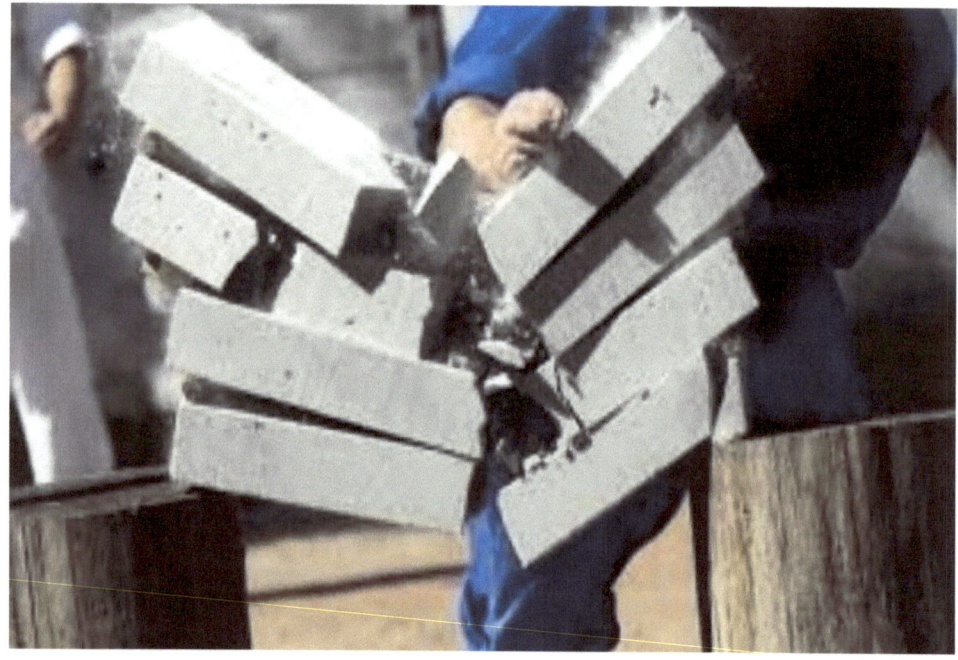

The other fact about unleashing your "True Inner Power" from your punches is your focus.

Staying focused on your target also plays a huge role, many fighters master the human body; which should have been your first step before trying this step. Why? Because once you master the human body, you can understand how much pain the body will take as well as how to focus your mind to execute this powerful attack like in the image you see here as well as focusing your power, you have to remember to shift almost all of your power into one single blow! That is the only way you'll be able to execute powerful blows like this image (below)

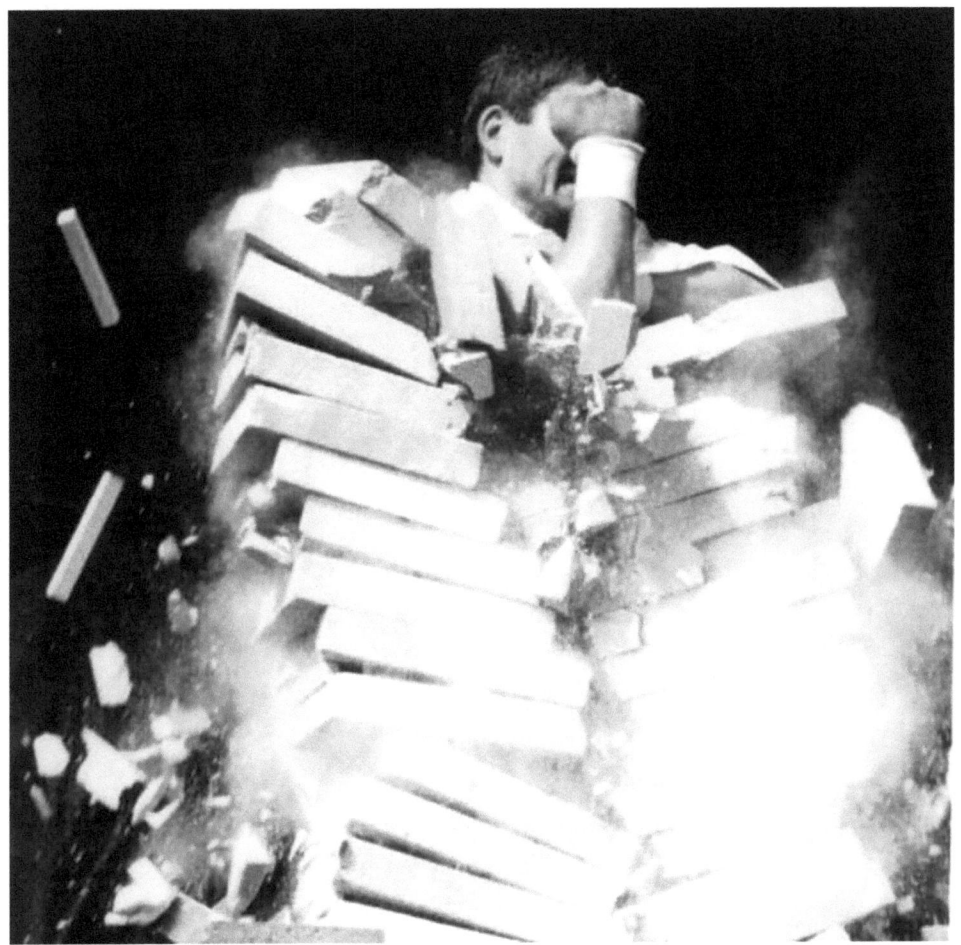

Remember: power shifting has to be mastered (After) focusing your power, & before (Focusing) your power, one needs to know how power & gravity goes "Hand-in-Hand"
But the biggest thing is understanding not to (fear) your task. Fear always cuts our power down at least 85%!!
Looking at something that seems impossible, will cause your body to weaken itself. Making your body (tissues) softer & more sensitive to hurting yourself, instead of releasing your power; you'll be doing the opposite.

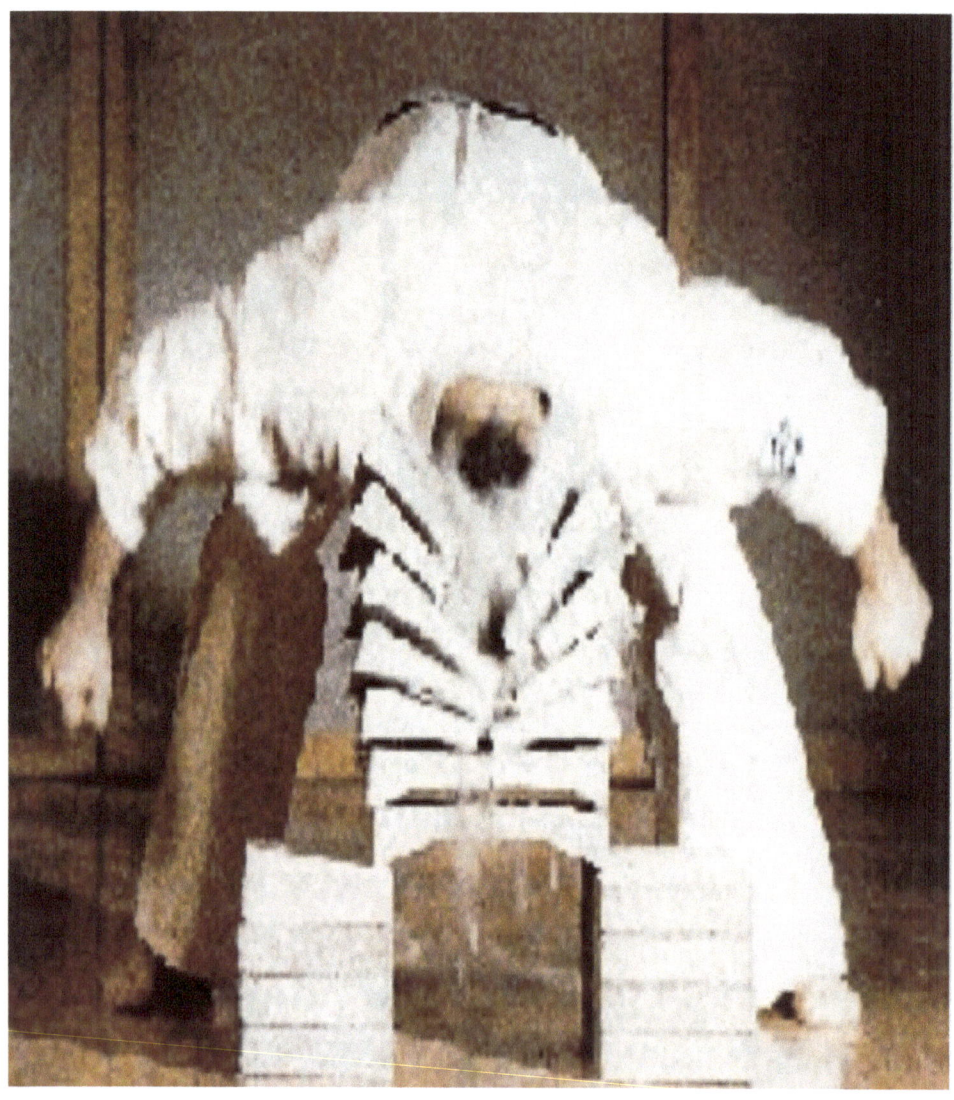

UNLOCKING
TRUE KICK
POWER

True kick power comes from the same training I explained from the "previous" sections of this book. True kicking power needs to be practiced every day as well as any other attacks. Performing an ultimate powerful kick like the ones in the images (Below) takes the other trainings, including different trainings like: yoga along with (Foot), (Leg) weights. This is the only way to unleash this kind of hidden leg power!

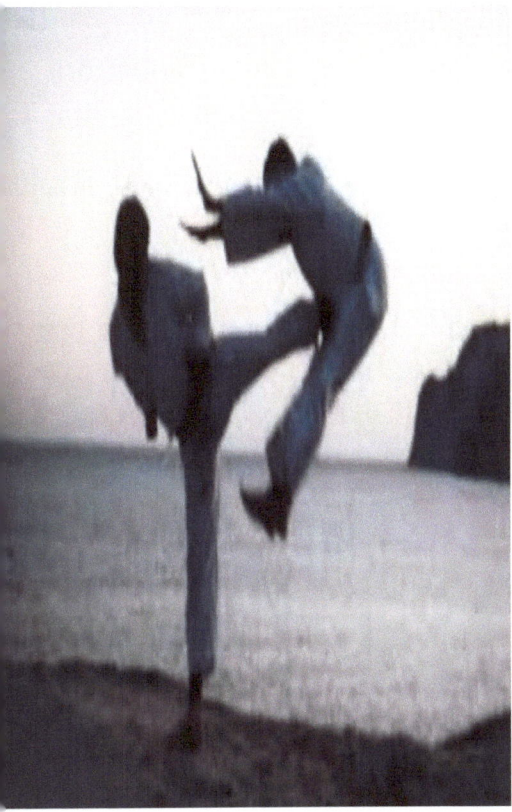
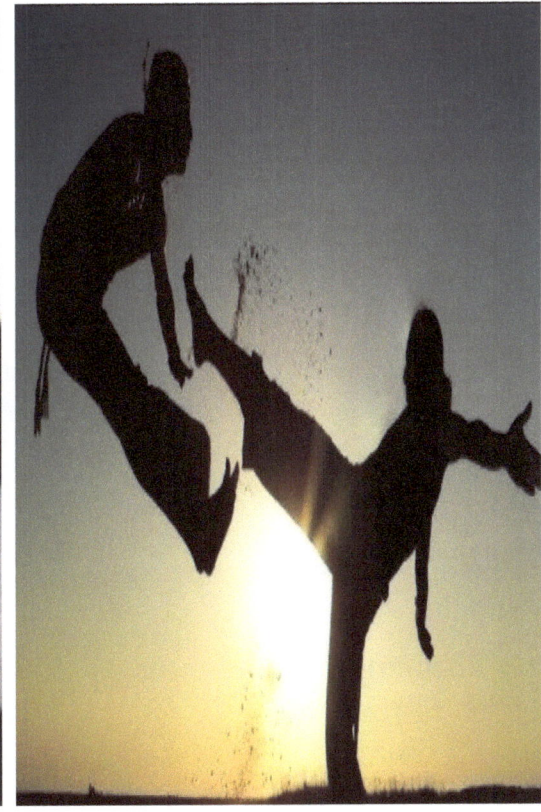

STEPS
TO
POWERFUL
KICKS

FIRST STEP:

Strength:

Now this is the hardest part of unleashing an ultra powerful kick. Leg strength has to be the main factor in performing this task. To build up leg strength, one has to practice (Kicking) hard objects so that the leg can get the feel of "Hard" materials. Try "Tapping" all parts of your foot against "bricks" or "steel" These will "toughen-up" your skin as well as giving your foot the advantage of feeling objects that are tougher than the human body itself.

SECOND STEP:

Speed:

Now on my previous sections I explained how to wear body weights, along with foot weights. In addition to these weights you'll need to train under water as well. Under water training, along with foot weights will help your feet get the speed they need to kick 2x as fast, & unleash 2x the power!!

THIRD STEP:

Focus:

Focusing on your strength & speed is Key to unlocking your true foot power! That's where (Yoga) comes in. Yoga stretching gives the body the relaxation it needs to be able to dig deep within itself to wanna unleash its full body power.

SURPASSING
OUR
POWER
LEVEL LIMITS

When it comes to "Surpassing" our normal inside power, one would have to toughen the (Inside) muscles. The inside muscles are our core strength. (Below) is a diagram of where our core strength power really lives. On the following pages ill explain how to train your body so it'll push itself to unleash its (un-normal) power potential.

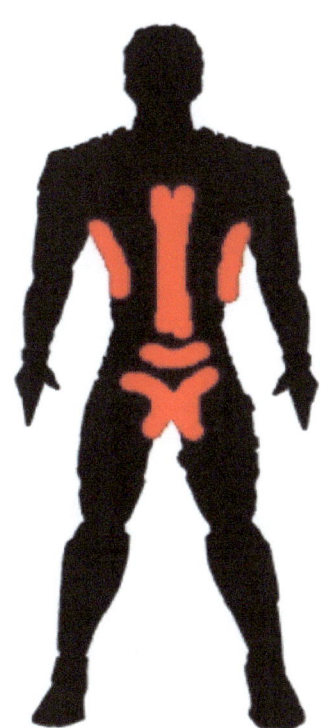

"INSIDE MUSCLES" are for:
- grounding
- balancing
- rotating
- pulling
- squeezing
- hardening
- generating power

Now to use these (Inner) body muscles, one needs to push the body beyond its normal limits!

I for one use "Parkour"

Parkour is a method of training your body & mind to overcome obstacles with speed & efficiency. However, the practice of Parkour also includes many challenges that need adaptability, creativity, & strategy. The main Key to remember when practicing (New) techniques with your body are to start off small, & slow. Like in the picture (Below) test your strength on average outside structures like a street sign pole or other obstacles. This will allow your body to get the feel of what kind of strength you already have, as well as what power you may need to unlock.

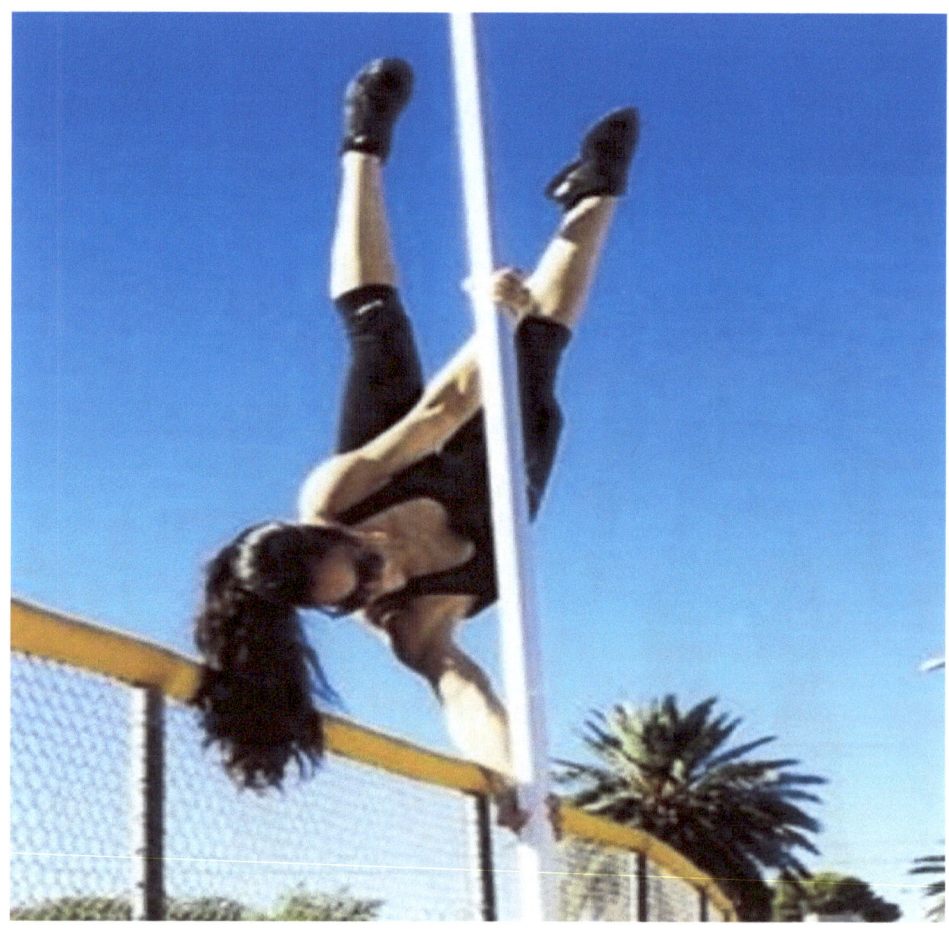

Once your body gets the feel of the small (Basic) obstacles, try "One-upping" your obstacles. Like in the pictures (Below)

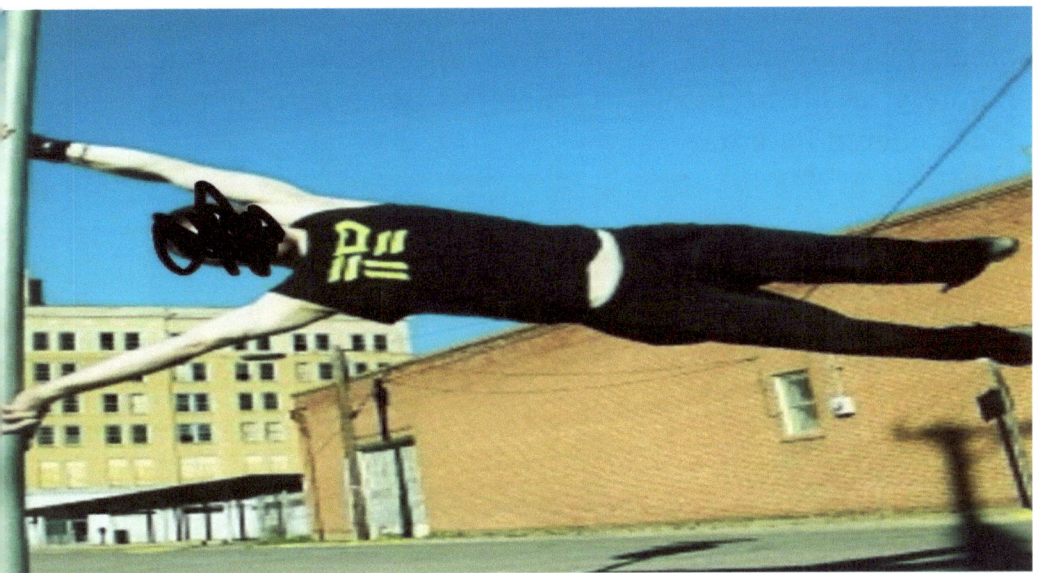

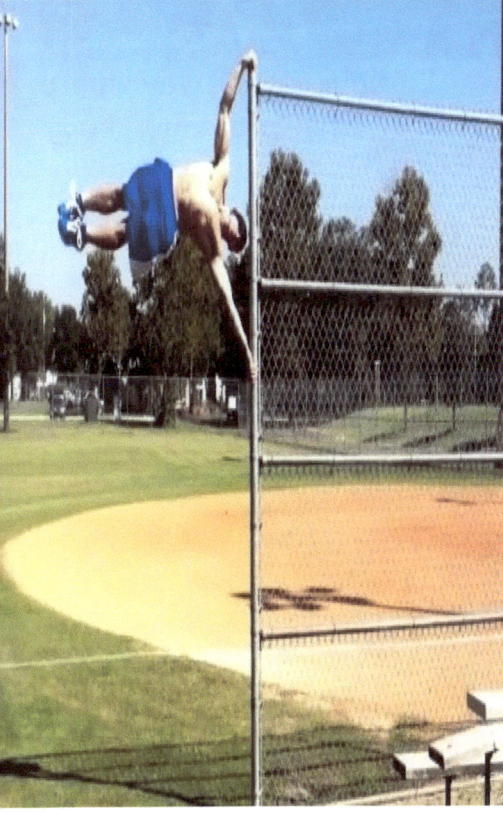

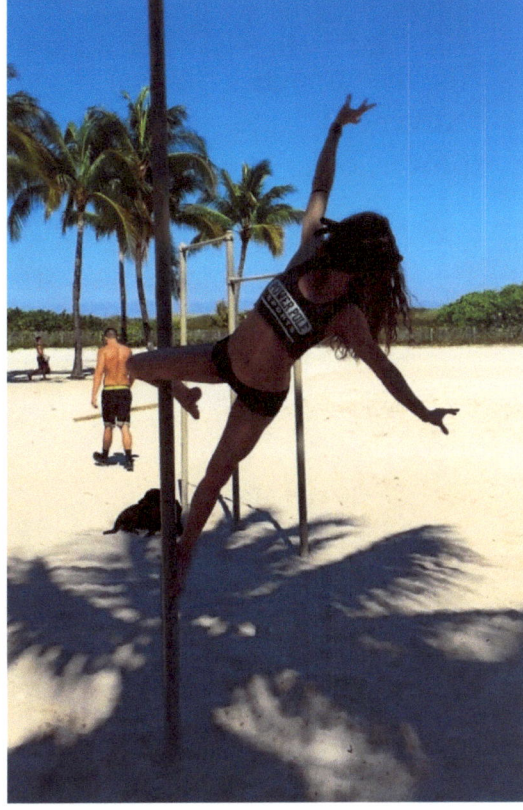

As a "Parkour" athlete, we are also known as tracers & traceuses, who use movements such as vaulting, running, climbing, swinging, & through obstacles. While Parkour can barrow movements from other disciplines, extraneous or purely aesthetic such as flips & twists are not typically considered Parkour.

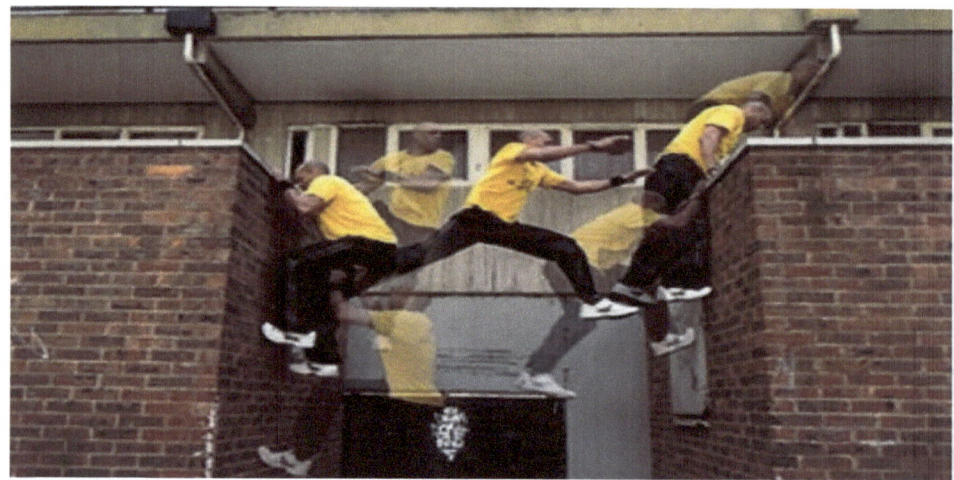

In the image (Below) it shows Parkour at a way more Advanced Rate. This is just a taste of what our inner body power looks like…once unleashed!

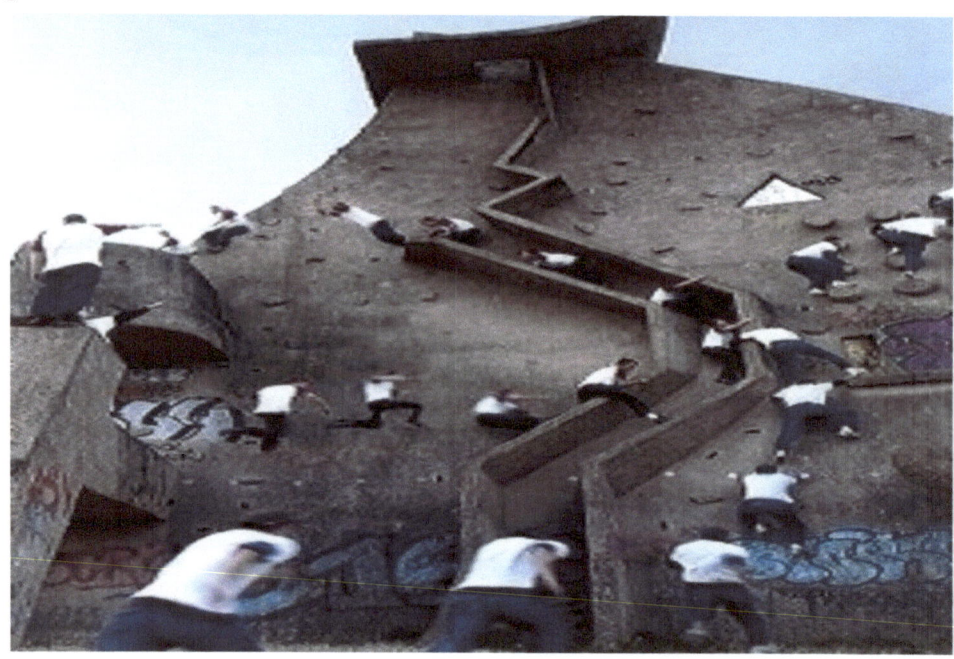

After lots of inner power body practicing, or (Parkour) training, here is what our human bodies will start to perform in a "Blink" of an eye!
These images are proof of what our speed, jumps, stamina, as well as body endurance is truly capable of!!

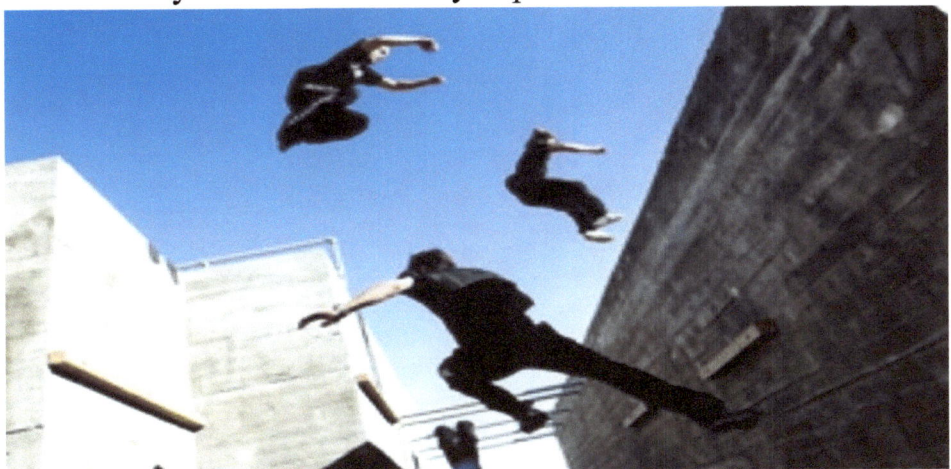

When your full body power is unleashed these will no long be obstacles…these will come naturally to you. (Mind over Matter) will cause this type of "Fear" to be over looked where it won't even apply to you as a person.

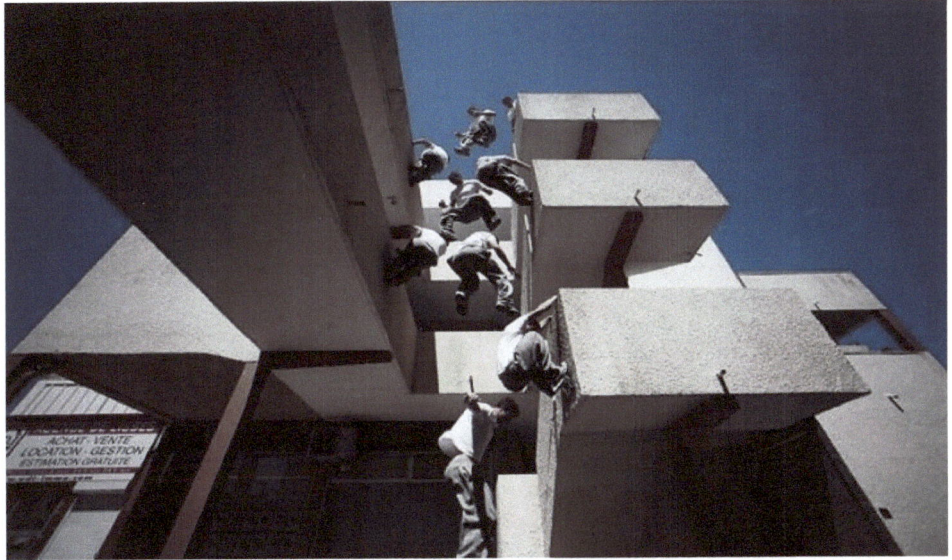

Its (Stunts) like these that the "average" human don't do! Im simply teaching you how to break that cycle.

To break the (Mind over Matter) cycle, all you have to do is try not to see your obstacle as an impossible task. Like in the images (Below) these power jumps may look impossible, but they truly are not.

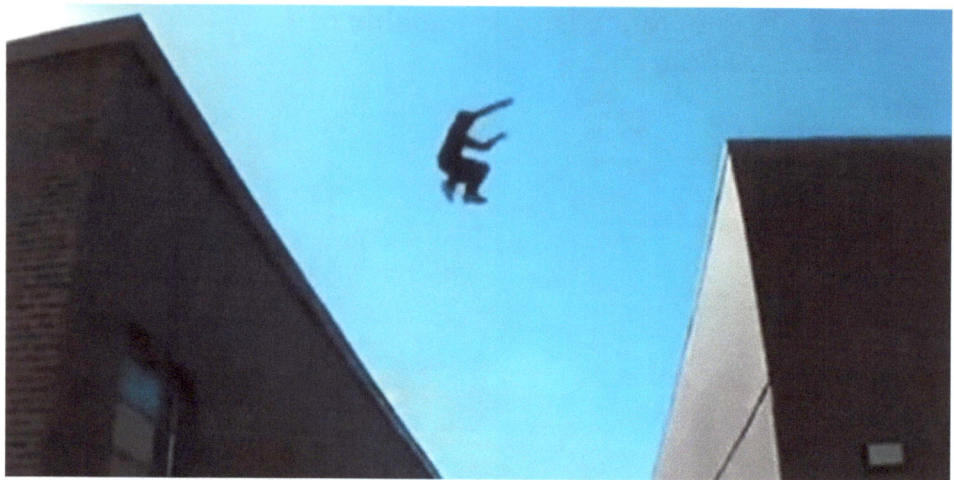

"Mind over matter", equals "Fear" being challenged. Separating the two, will always allow you to unleash this type of performance.

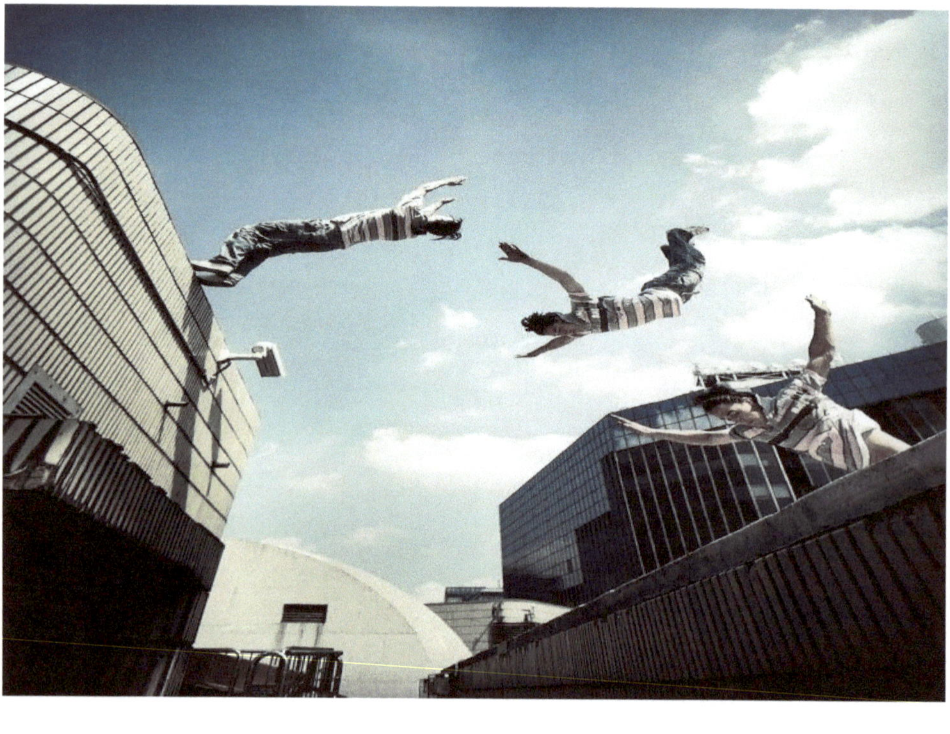

Always remember, the human body is an amazing instrument to be played in many different ways. Our body performances can "Astonishing" if we train our bodies.

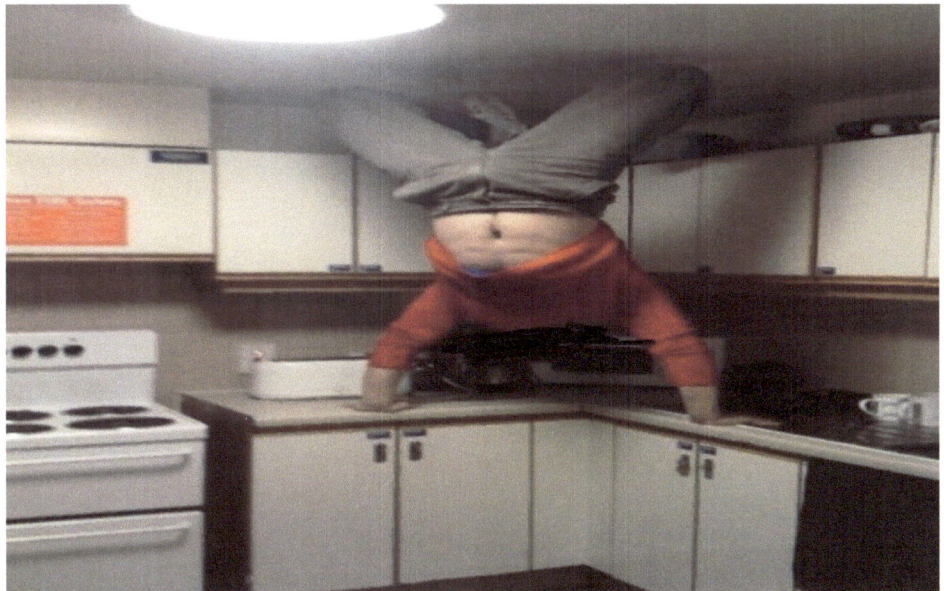

These images are just simple reminders of what kind of hidden power we all poses as humans. We just need a little practice.

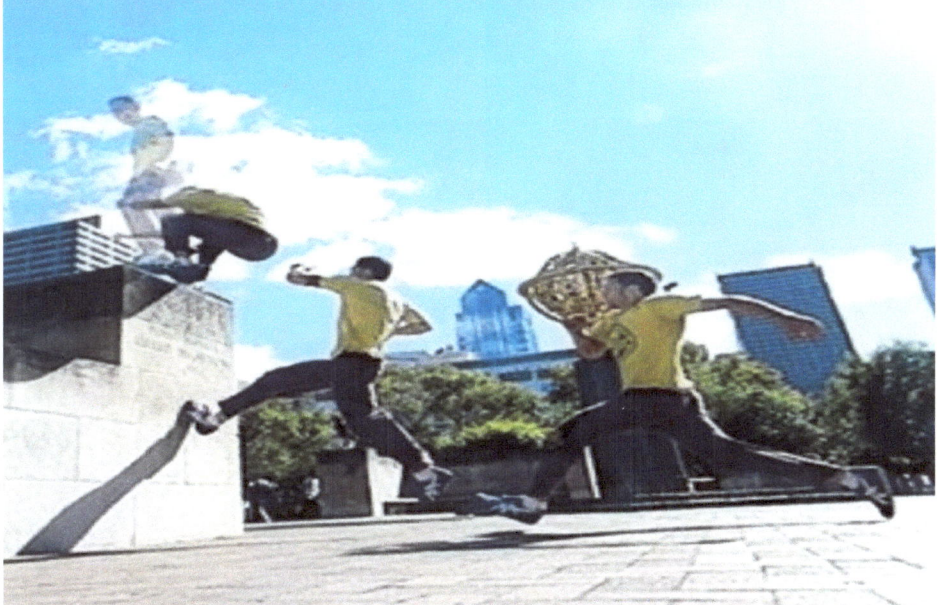

From (Kitchen hand-stands) to (Running up walls) it all can be done!.

Remember, all of our (Body-Senses) can be manipulated/ upgraded in amazing ways!
Inner power has to be triggered by (Self-Learning) & fear overcoming. Mastering the human body parts is crucial to all of these learning capabilities.

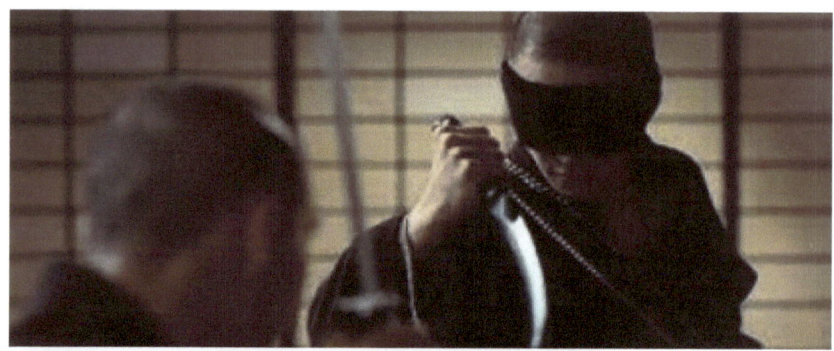

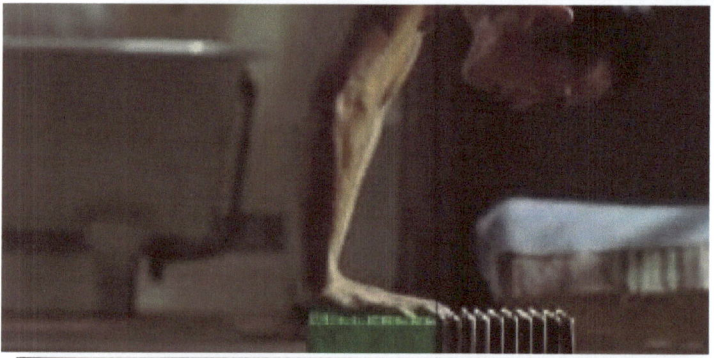

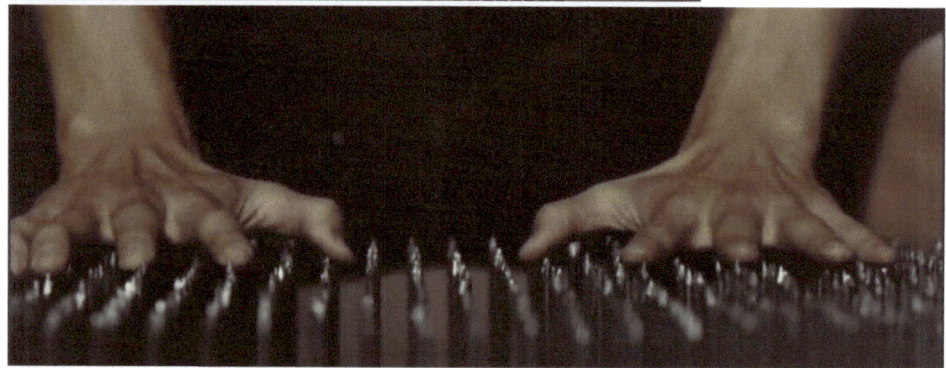

Even after being blind-folded; the human body can still "sense" where another human body is located. To do this technique, one needs to practice his or her main focusing skills. Great focus is keen, while motivating yourself to feel the air around yourself to feel their "vibrations" through their body.

PERSONAL NOTES

MEET THE AUTHOR

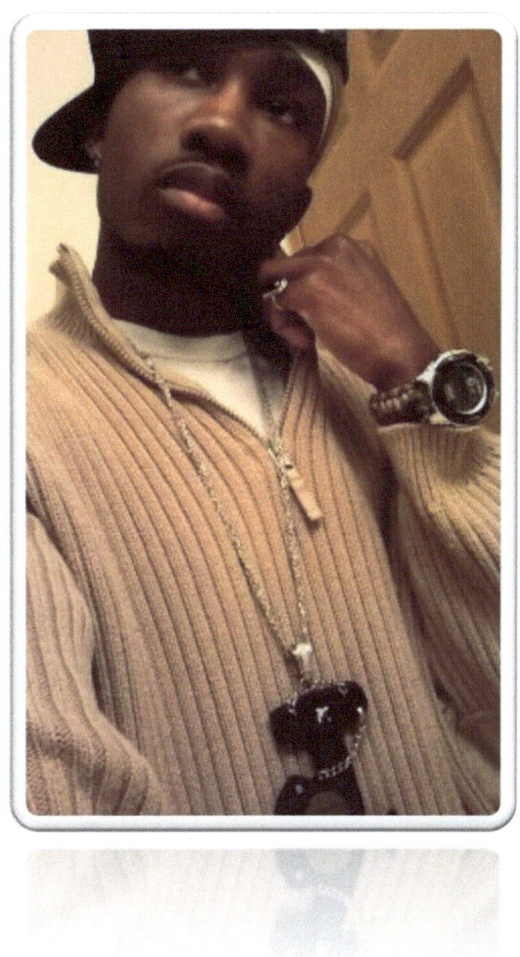

"JOHN LEE LOVE" is (author), & master inventor of "body-weaponry" who specializes in weapon mechanic body fusion, he is also Author of nineteen other publications which fifth teen of them are self-help guides for everyday life. He lives in Minneapolis Minnesota.